'Extraordinary and utterly co... ... ...
and part riveting history of the fateful and absorbing uncertainty
that is hypochondria, this book will be an illumination for
anyone who has ever wondered if they are ill.'

– **Adam Phillips, author of *On Giving Up***

'In *Hypochondria*, Will Rees pulls off an almost impossible
balancing act. He recalls his personal history with great clarity
and vulnerability, and he assembles a dazzling archive of his
fellow writers and hypochondriacs: Melville, Kafka, Freud,
Sartre, Didion. Hypochondria, Rees shows us, is a specific case
of fantasizing about what we cannot know – we are all, in our
own ways, hypochondriacs.'

– **Merve Emre, author of *The Personality Brokers***

'This elegant and finely crafted essay will be enlightening not
only for those who suffer from health anxieties but, more
generally, for anyone confronting the problem of inhabiting
the human body. Blending autobiography, history, and theory,
it raises crucial questions about our embodied existence in an
engaging and accessible way.'

– **Darian Leader, author of *The New Black:
Mourning, Melancholia and Depression***

'I marvelled at this elegant and intellectually capacious book.
Unmoored by its elusive subject, Rees innovates an utterly
engrossing mode of inquiry that seems forged from the very
material of hypochondria itself – radical doubt. And, like all

good hypochondriacs, this book is many things at once: a philosophical intrigue, a meticulous catalogue of symptoms, a literature of writerly ailments, and a gripping tale of desire's shadow. Here are hypochondria's many indignities, but also its raptures and romance. What emerges from Rees's ability to dwell in uncertainty is proof of doubt's generative potential; its questions are insistent and hard-won vital signs. What if we are what we read? What if health is little more than blissful ignorance? What if we can never be sure of just how sick we really are?'

– **Daisy Lafarge, author of** *Paul*

'*Hypochondria* is a beautifully written, exacting, exquisite piece of literature and an urgent intervention into a deeply necessary conversation that has languished in the shadows for far too long. This book is as clever as it is brave, and it will change and move everyone who reads it. To capture the intricacies of our relationship with illness, both individually and in our collective consciousness, is one of the most difficult things a writer can do – Rees has done it perfectly. Everyone must read this book.'

– **Lucia Osborne-Crowley, author of** *The Lasting Harm*

HYPOCHONDRIA

WILL REES

COACH HOUSE BOOKS, TORONTO

first edition

LIBRARY AND ARCHIVES CANADA CATALOGUING IN PUBLICATION

Title: Hypochondria / Will Rees.
Names: Rees, Will, author.
Description: First edition.
Identifiers: Canadiana 20240443675 | ISBN 9781552454848 (softcover)
Subjects: LCSH: Rees, Will—Mental health. | LCSH: Illness anxiety disorder—
Patients—Biography. | LCSH: Illness anxiety disorder in literature. | LCGFT:
Autobiographies.
Classification: LCC RC552.H8 R44 2025 | DDC 616.85/250092—dc23

Hypochondria is available as an ebook: ISBN 978 1 77056 823 5 (EPUB), ISBN
978 1 77056 824 2 (PDF)

Purchase of the print version of this book entitles you to a free digital copy.
To claim your ebook of this title, please email sales@chbooks.com with proof
of purchase. (Coach House Books reserves the right to terminate the free
digital download offer at any time.)

The events described here happened more than a decade ago. Today I look back, bemused, and write about 'hypochondria.' This is a story I am telling. A true one, I hope.

SUSPENDED IN DARKNESS

Throughout my adolescence and into my mid-twenties I spent a lot of time trying to acquire knowledge about my body, never permitting myself to accept the vague blend of supposition and wishful thinking that was widely available and with which, unaccountably, others appeared to be satisfied. I was unwell, that much was certain. The question of how was one to which I applied myself studiously. Of course, I had theories. Looking back, these tended to change quite frequently, and yet the fear was always the same: in short, that I was dying, that I had some dreadful and no doubt painful disease that, for all my worrying, I had carelessly allowed to reach the point beyond which it would now have become incurable. My researches required me to enlist the help of doctors. Above all, I sought a scan that would light up every region of my body, that would reveal, clearly and distinctly, what was the matter with it. To my mind a scan had come to represent complete and perfect knowledge – no more secrets.

'The position of hypochondria is still suspended in darkness.' This was the candid assessment of Sigmund Freud at a meeting of the Vienna Psychoanalytic Society. By 1909 Freud was a successful psychiatrist whose disciples credited him with having put psychology onto a scientific footing, and with having unlocked the secrets of another, closely related ancient malady, hysteria. His colleagues proposed they celebrate the march of progress, the steady inroads they had made into the darkest recesses of the soul, by producing a pamphlet that would inform the medical community about the accomplishments of their new science. Agreeing to this idea, Freud nevertheless insisted that his colleagues would have to be transparent about 'the limits of our knowledge,' foremost among which, he said, was their failure to elucidate the nature of hypochondria.

A few years later, in 1912, little seemed to have changed. Freud wrote in a letter to his friend Sándor Ferenczi that the 'darkness' surrounding hypochondria was 'a great disgrace to our efforts.' For all his attempts, Freud had come up with no definite understanding of the condition, only 'supposition.' It was as if Freud were suggesting that, for all his colleagues' chatter about progress, little had changed in the three hundred years since Robert Burton sat down to compose his vast and never-completed *Anatomy of Melancholy*, in which he wrote that hypochondria's 'symptoms are so ambiguous' that 'physicians cannot determine of the part affected.'

According to the humoral medicine that held sway from ancient Greece until the eighteenth century, 'hypochondria' named a physical disease that was seated in the abdomen, in an area called the hypochondrium. This put gastrointestinal complaints at the centre of its symptomatology. Burton, for instance, includes among the symptoms of 'windy Hypochondriacal Melancholy' such visceral discomforts as 'sharp belchings, fulsome crudities, heat in the bowels, wind and rumbling in the guts, [and] vehement gripings.' For the learned Oxonian, however, it was hypochondria's tendency to generate 'fear and sorrow' that made it terrible and fascinating. Over the years these qualities increasingly came to predominate.

Today, we recognize (or think we recognize) hypochondria to be a psychological condition. Present-day hypochondriacs are sometimes treated with talking therapy, occasionally with antidepressants, and most commonly of all with contempt.

On its winding journey from unhealthy hypochondrium to unsound mind, much of what is named by the word 'hypochondria' has been altered beyond recognition: the condition's centuries-long association with excessive flatulence, for instance, vanished in the nineteenth century; meanwhile, fears about illness came increasingly to the fore, ultimately eclipsing all other symptoms.

However, one thing that has remained consistent is the confusion it provokes among diagnosticians, the crises of categorization; even today a professional debate continues as to whether hypochondria is best described as a primary or a secondary disorder, an illness or a symptom – or whether, indeed, it is a clinical entity at all. In 2013 the American Psychiatric Association (APA) removed hypochondriasis from the fifth edition of its *Diagnostic and Statistical Manual* (DSM), replacing it with two distinct but overlapping diagnoses: somatic symptom disorder and illness anxiety disorder – two conditions that, although very similar, sit on completely separate illness spectrums. If the letters pages of the *British Medical Journal* are anything to go by, the move has generated a lot of confusion, leaving many physicians unsure of where to place erstwhile hypochondriacs. In practice many have retained the diagnosis which, it is important to note, is still to be found in the World Health Organization's 2019 eleventh edition of the *International Classification of Diseases* (ICD).

The position of hypochondria has never been less certain. Perhaps we can simply say that hypochondria appears destined to trouble the medical imagination: neither fully mental nor physical, not quite disease and yet hardly 'health.'

*

Being suspended in darkness means not having the ground beneath one's feet. It entails a total loss of any meaningful sense of up or down, left or right, so that one does not even know forward from back, a straight line from a circle. The position that Freud is describing is that of being over an abyss. In this sense he might be thought to have been speaking not only about the position of hypochondria, but about that of the *hypochondriac.* I can think of no better way to describe the lightless place in which hypochondriacs find themselves, their desire for some definite and illuminating understanding that pushes them to grasp, anxiously, at the very limits of their knowledge. What impels the hypochondriac is, above all, a desire to know their body – to know that it is healthy, to know that it is free from disease. And yet, equivocal and iterative, hypochondria not only activates but undermines our fantasies of complete understanding.

'There is scarce any thing that hath not killed somebody,' wrote John Donne in 1623, 'a hair, a feather hath done it; nay, that which is our best antidote against it hath done it; the best cordial hath been deadly poison.' There are people who can construe any situation as a scene of danger, who constantly ask 'what if?' I was never really like that. Fear for me was reductive, not accretive. Always, it came down to the same old story: a cancer that, wherever it had first arisen, had quietly run its course through my entire body. This went on for many years, during which there were leads and breakthroughs, though generally I moved in circles. What was more, even as my fears reached a crescendo, I could never quite shake the suspicion that I was simply making it all up.

This began when I was at university. I was studying literature and philosophy, but I spent just as much time browsing medical sites, spending long nights alone at my laptop. Each time I had a new symptom I'd enter it into Google, which never failed to produce the dismal result.

Sitting in hospital waiting rooms or lying in bed, I would picture the appalling things due to happen to me – images that must have been pulled together from different sources: TV, newspapers, things overheard, misremembered, combined, distorted. 'Having always lived in fear of being surprised by the worst,' writes Emil Cioran, 'I have tried in every circumstance to get a head start, flinging myself into misfortune long before it occurred.' For me this was not fatalism, however. Fundamentally, it was optimistic: if I could picture it, vividly and exactly, then forecast would become fantasy and by that token would be prevented from coming to pass.

During those years, fear was not a stable quantity. There were times of acute crisis, times when I had no life outside of waiting for test results, no future beyond the horizon of the bad news that I expected, at any moment, to receive. Other times fear was only a background hum, more annoyance than affliction, like the distant traffic sound one hears only when, wanting to be irritated, one turns an ear toward it. These periods of remission never lasted. When they ended, I scolded myself for my complacency and resolved to commit myself whole-heartedly to my fears.

And yet it is important to say that throughout all this I remained outwardly 'normal,' a rank-and-file member of what, in *On Being Ill*, Virginia Woolf calls the 'army of the upright.' Susan Sontag describes illness as 'the night-side of life.' My fears fell in with this diurnal rhythm. I suppose this was a sort of compromise, a way of continuing to invest in a life that, even at my darkest moments, I knew I might end up having to live. During the day, I carried on as usual. I went to class, later to work. I colluded like anyone else in the open secret of mortality, performing all those little tasks and rituals on which any person who had frankly acknowledged Death would flatly refuse to spend his quota of minutes. When I bought shoes, I bought sturdy ones to last. I separated card and plastic and put my bottles in the bin labelled BOTTLES. I made plans for the future, my CV was always up to date. But at night, my mind was constantly drawn back to that other reality, to that dreadful, hidden truth that was waiting to be brought to light.

*

This book covers a five-year period of my life, which began at a time when I was convinced that I had a brain tumour, and ended in my mid-twenties, by which point this had quietly morphed into the belief that I had lymphoma. These two moments, these two periods of crisis when the question of health hung darkest over my everyday, bookend *Hypochondria*, which also looks at the history of this condition, and at those who have attempted to understand it. Along the way, I write about other people who have been preoccupied with their health, doing so with an evident, if not entirely justified bias toward those who have left behind the most eloquent and comprehensive paper trails regarding their phantom fears – which of course is to say, writers.

Some of these people referred to themselves as hypochondriacs, while others didn't. Even among those who did apply this word to their own experience, exactly what they meant, the precise nature of the suffering they hoped to name with it, varied considerably. In writing about these historical figures, I'm not going to be making any retrospective diagnoses of 'hypochondriasis' – a harmless enough pastime for retired doctors, I suppose, but not of much genuine interest. In fact it doesn't matter to me whether these figures were 'really' hypochondriac (or anxious, depressed, suffering from an undiagnosed post-viral condition) for the reason that hypochondria, I will be suggesting, is a diagnosis that puts into question how certain we can ever be about *any* diagnosis – including, needless to say, a diagnosis of hypochondria. Call it what you will; it's the uncertainty that interests me, not the labels with which we try to contain it.

Lastly, writing about hypochondria, my own and others', means writing about what didn't happen, or doesn't seem to have happened; it means recording what is nearly nothing. At times this nothing has constituted the larger part of my life. For years I trained my eyes on it. Gradually, it revealed itself to be wavering and various; it flickered and shifted, it wouldn't stay still. It's true that I was probably more stuck on it than most, but it's also true that what is nothing, or nearly nothing, exerts a pressure on even the most grounded existence: it could be a lie you live, a fear, a dream, a plan that doesn't come to fruition and that perhaps was not ever intended to. What doesn't exist, or barely exists, might have an overbearing presence in your daily life, or it might occupy it more minimally, like a name you can't quite remember, like a tune that haunts your inner ear.

How can we get to know these aspects of our lives? Common sense invites us to turn away from them, to dismiss them as trivial, which in a certain sense they are. In this book I take a different approach. With his famous practice of 'evenly suspended attention,' Freud advised psychoanalysts to bracket the usual hierarchies of significance when interpreting the patient's experience. Whenever one 'select[s] from the material before him,' he warned, 'he is in danger of never finding anything but what he already knows.' What Freud advocates for here is a method of reading in which analysts refuse to discriminate in advance between truth and fiction, reality and delusion, the important and the trivial, thereby opening themselves to the possibility of being surprised out of their habitual ways of thinking, finding what they did not already know.

If Freud is present in these pages more often than may be widely preferred, it is not because any of his (quite unsatisfying) theories of hypochondria. It's because better than anyone else he understood that uncertainty is not always a problem to be solved. This is something that the French writer Maurice Blanchot is suggesting when he writes that literature calls upon 'the resources of our ignorance,' as if to say that reading, however diligent, however careful and attentive, always involves an experience of not-knowing – the space for rereading. It is to be reconfronted by this basic fact that, time and again, I find myself returning to psychoanalysis and literature.

In his analysis of the hypochondriacal German judge Daniel Paul Schreber, Freud was famously surprised to observe a similarity between Schreber's baroque fantasies and his own psychoanalytic theories. Nevertheless, Freud resisted the impulse to clear things up, saying that it 'remains for the future to decide whether there is more delusion in my theory than I should like to admit, or whether there is more truth in Schreber's delusion that other people are as yet prepared to believe.' Before proceeding, let's pause to note that this is always a risk with hypochondria: that the person who seeks to cast light on it will instead find themselves being led into the dark.

LOOMINGS

One day in 2010, I got a headache. The pain was not severe, but it was constant – accompanied by a strange feeling of belatedness which meant that, when I first became conscious of it, I knew it had already been going on for some time, lingering just beneath the threshold of awareness. How long exactly, I couldn't say – weeks, definitely. Maybe it had been years.

After about a month I visited the doctor. In those days, this was not a knee-jerk response. This must have been at the start of June because it was warm out, and I remember that I was on my way to return a suitcase and two shopping bags full of overdue library books – something that, to my discredit, I did only twice a year, on the first Monday after the end of the winter and the summer terms.

The doctor had an earnest, warbling, confident way of speaking that, in spite of her evident commitment to the tenets of mainstream medicine, gave her the unshakeable air of an alternative healer. She explained that what I was experiencing were called tension headaches, an ailment that was common among students and during exam season practically universal. I said that I didn't feel very tense. The doctor asked whether the pain felt like a tightness across both sides of the head. A kind of squeezing? Like an elastic band being pulled tight? Like a fist clenching around your skull? I said that it did not feel like these things. Yes, she said, nodding meaningfully. Every person experiences tension differently.

The doctor asked me what medication I'd been using to manage the pain. I was thrown by this question; the thought had not occurred to me. This was, in many ways, quite surprising, since I have never been a person to make a virtue out of forbearance and actually consider my tolerance to pain to be less developed than the average. In the case of this headache, however, my attitude was edging closer to that of Franz Kafka. A century earlier, the writer told his soon-to-be fiancée Felice Bauer that he never took aspirin because doing so, he said, created 'a sense of artificiality' that in his opinion was far worse than any 'natural affliction.' Aspirin had been developed a few years earlier in the laboratories of the Bayer Company. Originally intended to treat rheumatism, it quickly gained popularity among healthy consumers looking to ease the ordinary pains of modern living. However, for Kafka it was vital to pay attention to every aspect of one's existence, no matter how small or seemingly trivial; which was why, as he later said, he made a habit of viewing his life through 'microscopical eyes.' As Kafka explained to Felice, if you had a headache, you had to undergo the experience of pain and treat it as a sign, before examining your entire life, right down to its most minute detail, 'so as to understand where the origins of your headaches are hidden.'

The idea of taking painkillers struck me as irresponsible, even reckless, like disconnecting a fire alarm because it has interrupted your sleep. Besides, the pain itself was bearable. Only its persistence concerned me, the meaning of it. Like Kafka, I wanted to understand the headache. The doctor told me to come back in a few weeks if things hadn't got better, sooner if they got worse. I left her office holding a bottle of aspirin, which I promptly deposited in the bin.

*

In her short essay 'In Bed,' Joan Didion writes about the chronic headaches that she suffered from on a weekly basis. Didion begins by explaining that migraine is an inherited condition, a 'physiological error.' By the end of the essay, however, Didion is describing a sly complicity between the migraine and its sufferer:

> We have reached a certain understanding, my migraine and I. It never comes when I am in real trouble … It comes instead when I am fighting not an open but a guerrilla war with my own life, during weeks of small household confusions, lost laundry, unhappy help, canceled appointments, on days when the telephone rings too much and I get no work done and the wind is coming up.

The migraines that regularly kept Didion hauled up in bed appear to be an unbearable yet not entirely unwelcome remission from the aching responsibilities of everyday life. And in this sense, a sort of pain relief.

My headache was nothing like that. My headache was very bearable. Terribly bearable. So that instead of extricating me from my everyday life, it pushed me deeper into it. I became irascible, morose. My entire life came to resemble one of those days when the wind is coming up; one of those days when in answer to the question 'what's wrong?' we are obliged, through gritted teeth, to answer 'nothing' so as to spare ourselves the graver indignity of uttering 'everything.'

As summer wore on I occasionally noticed myself not noticing the headache. I might be swimming, or making love, or reading, and it would happily occur to me that I no longer felt any pain. However, this reflection always served to drive it out of hiding, and the mild, negligible pain would resume its place at the forefront of my mind. These were not spells of remission, therefore, so much as lapses of attention. As time passed, they became fewer and farther between.

By autumn I had started noticing lots of other little anomalies. I became forgetful. Words kept escaping me. In a crowded bar one evening, I spent fifteen minutes trying to guess where I'd met the bespectacled, aloof young man in front of me, certain that he was playing a game, not letting on. Until, annoyed and frankly a little unnerved, he finally said, 'Look, I'm just trying to get a drink.' I developed a twitch in my left eye, which would refer down to my middle finger, so that in lectures I always seemed to be tapping out the unsteady beat to some inaudible tune. One pupil became slightly larger than the other and coffee started tasting weird and metallic. One morning I turned on the tap and had no idea whether the water was hot or cold.

I developed a very mild but persistent case of the hiccups, just one, two, maybe three solitary little hiccups each day. Can hiccups be caused by brain cancer? I asked Google. Yes, it answered – if it is advanced. Sometime later, or earlier, I started to smell things that didn't seem to have any external source. Burning, usually. Other times the astringent, chemical smell of VHS cleaner, a substance whose existence I had not considered for more than a decade. One morning I woke up and my nostrils were filled with the indescribable scent of the villa in Spain where as a child I spent my long, dull, lovely summers.

My eyesight, which had always been perfect, began to flare at the edges, as though there were always something flickering just outside my field of vision. I would turn suddenly, trying to catch it; at which point it would cease, recommencing as soon as I turned back around. Later it became grainy, like a poorly tuned television, although only when I looked at empty spaces like the sky or the ceiling: details I could see perfectly, it was the absences that escaped me, becoming present. At night I would hear a sound; it was quiet at first, barely perceptible, but over time it became louder and more complex as my ears gradually attuned themselves to its frequency.

At some point I started keeping a list of all these things as they arose, doing so on a loose sheet of paper headed SYMPTOMS, which I stowed in my sock drawer. Reading back over that list, it struck me that it resembled the descriptions of illnesses that I browsed online. This was the first time I had written about myself. Like later attempts, this modest venture into diarizing was intended to clarify my experience, and in this regard the habit was successful. But it was precisely for this reason that I also felt it was distorting things, lending them clear outlines that, in reality, they rarely had.

And even now I feel there is the risk in setting all this down on paper that it will give weight and solidity to a set of experiences whose most maddening quality, as I recall it, was their shimmering insubstantiality. It's true that there were times when these phenomena occurred simultaneously, times when they condensed into something like a palpable disease. Or at the risk of putting things a little dramatically, when these sensory glitches had seeped so deeply into my experience of the world that, as I once explained to a friend, it felt as if reality itself was becoming sick. However, these periods were punctuated by spells of relative calm. Days would pass by without incident, perhaps when I was busy, happily industrious, unconsciously embedded in life. But in a pattern that was becoming familiar, no sooner would I reflect on the absence of these disturbances than I would start to notice them again.

You could say that my attention was producing these things; you could say it was revealing them.

A SERIOUS, SCHOLARLY STUDY

A few years ago, I decided to write a history of hypochondria, a serious, scholarly study that would diligently chart its development, from the humoral theories of Hippocrates and Galen to Freudian metapsychology and on to its current position after its banishment from the DSM. It had been some time since my own health had been a concern to me. And though things were never quite cleared up, in the intervening years hypochondria had become the lens through which I fondly viewed my old fears – which led me to feel there was a sort of justness, and no little pleasure, in regarding the fact that it would now become the object of my first piece of historical scholarship.

I was not a historian, so I asked an academic research body to fund a PhD. It turned out that little had been written on hypochondria. This made it relatively easy to make the case that I would be providing the required 'original contribution to knowledge,' a phrase that summoned in me the Babelian fantasy of a vast tome, an ever-expanding ledger at the bottom of which I would shortly be adding my name. Soon, and with greater ease than I'd expected, I was enthusiastically applying myself to the task of becoming a historian by producing my serious, scholarly study of hypochondria.

This was at the end of 2019. Over the course of that winter I occasionally saw an article about the novel coronavirus that was spreading through the east of China. By the beginning of March everyone was worrying about illness and wiping door handles and washing their hands ten times a day. What happens to hypochondria, I found myself wondering, in a world in which every surface, and even the air around us, has become a potential vector of disease? Had we now, all of us, become hypochondriacs? Or as an old joke goes, had the entire world discovered that the secret cure for hypochondria is … illness?

Events seemed to be lending my project a certain timeliness. On the other hand, in the face of a very real pandemic, my research into imaginary illness had never seemed more negligible. I really can't account for it, but that spring, as I moved my life online, adjusting myself to those times that were widely reported to be unprecedented, I found myself stalked by the strangest feeling of déjà vu. With little else to do, I threw myself into my work. On certain days this work felt vital; on others it felt absurd. Much of the time it felt as though I was doing nothing at all, simply sitting at home, browsing old medical books on my laptop, basically just making things up.

*

In his 1916 *First Contributions to Psycho-analysis*, Sándor Ferenczi quotes from the diary of one of his patients: 'Hypochondria surrounds my soul like a fine mist, or rather like a cobweb, just as a fungus covers a swamp.' Hardly successful from a literary perspective, the description is nevertheless striking in how its uneasy mix of metaphors fail to come together to form a stable image. In doing so they give expression to a shapeshifting condition that constantly gnaws at the edges of language, flickering into view and back out again, demanding while refusing to avail itself to description. What begins for Ferenczi's patient as a fine mist quickly darkens: 'Man surely is not here to be veiled in such a cobweb, suffocated, and robbed of the light of the sun.' Hypochondria, as described by these discordant strange images, is opaque, impenetrable, but also airy and gossamer-like, nearly inexistent.

As the world plunged into a full-blown health crisis, it was hypochondria's proximity to nothingness that came to strike me as its most defining feature. It isn't just that the feared illness might not exist. Despite having once named a 'real' bodily disease, during the last century and a half the word *hypochondria* has itself come to refer to a kind of negativity, a scepticism that is scrupulously, perhaps ruinously, attuned to the gaps in medicine's knowledge of the body.

'Hypochondria is the only illness I don't have,' the comedian Tony Hancock used to joke, playing on its status as a fear of illness that is also a form of illness. Hypochondria, as I was coming to see it, is always a two-faced condition. On the one hand it names a long-standing medical diagnosis, an object of positivist medical knowledge. Yet at some point it also started to name something else, harder to pin down – a form of doubt, a style of interpretation.

To be caught in the web of hypochondria is to enter into an altered relationship to language in which words cease to produce certainties, only questions. What does this headache mean? Is something wrong with me? Am I sick? Am I dying? How can I be sure that I am well? Can I ever be sure? Or is certainty the very thing that must be given up if I want to feel well? In which case is health ever anything more than a feeling? And therefore, perhaps, an illusion?

These are the escalating questions the hypochondriac insistently asks, and while they're easily dismissed, they're a lot more difficult to answer. Like the child's, the hypochondriac's incessant questioning reveals painful gaps in the stories we tell about ourselves and about the world. No wonder we dislike them. No sooner have we admitted such questions into consideration than we find ourselves forced to reckon with how little we really know, with just how much wilful ignorance and wishful thinking are involved in what typically goes by the name of 'health.'

*

'He can neither believe, nor be comfortable in his unbelief.'
Nathaniel Hawthorne was writing here of his friend Herman
Melville, though I prefer to think he was summarizing a more
general plight, that of those consigned to view the world through
the lens of hypochondria, with its uneasy blend of doubt and
fear, its thwarted desire for the sustaining illusion. Whatever
way you look at it, hypochondria is a question of belief. Being a
hypochondriac means refusing to believe the mounting evidence
that one is well. Or (which might amount to the same) it means
wishing more than anything to believe in one's health and therefore searching for irrefutable evidence in support of it.

Throughout his whole adult life Melville suffered from what
he called 'Blue devils, hypochondria, and doleful dumps.' In
the opening lines of *Moby-Dick*, published five years before
Hawthorne's diagnosis, Melville had gone so far as to elevate
this condition to the novel's prime mover:

> ... and especially whenever my hypos get such an upper
> hand of me, that it requires a strong moral principle to
> prevent me from deliberately stepping into the street,
> and methodically knocking people's hats off – then, I
> account it high time to get to sea as soon as I can.

It's in another seafaring tale that we really get a sense of what
hypochondria meant for Melville. In *Benito Cereno*, Captain
Delano, 'a man ... incapable of satire or irony,' boards a ship
captained by the saturnine and mistrustful Don Cereno, a fellow
traveller of 'those hypochondriacs, Johnson and Byron.' Before
long, Cereno's infernal doubting infects the Delano like a

'contagion' so that, prey to 'strange questions' and 'passing from one suspicious thing to another,' the earnest American slides into a Cartesian vortex from which he is unable to discern truth from error ('if I could only be certain that, in my uneasiness, my senses did not deceive me'). In the pressurized atmosphere of the text, these doubts infect the reader, too, who quickly finds themselves implicated in this game of guessing and second-guessing. So, with Melville we might say: once hypochondria has entered the scene, it is *everyone's* equilibrium that risks being ruffled.

A person can 'feel well … but he can never know that he is healthy,' Immanuel Kant once wrote, thereby proposing an incommensurability between health and knowledge that, for some people, can be difficult to swallow. To be a hypochondriac, in the words of James Boswell, means succumbing to a 'universal scepticism.' Or as Gilles Deleuze puts it in his essay about Melville, to 'a negativism beyond all negation.' If these statements are correct, then far from being a discrete and bounded object of positive knowledge, 'hypochondria' would seem to name a corrosive force that dissolves our claims to know anything at all – not only a limit to, but the very other of knowledge.

This is what Freud was grappling with, too, when he complained that the position of hypochondria was 'still' suspended in darkness: he was pointing out that he was living in an age of medical enlightenment, an age that had successfully unlocked the secrets of countless bodily diseases and which, under his guidance, was beginning to unlock the secrets of the soul. And yet for all that, hypochondria remained beyond grasp. As if, in an age that had illuminated body and soul, hypochondria had come to name, not an illness as such, but rather whatever had not yet been brought to light – the haunting spectre of uncertainty that remained, still, just beyond the reach of medical knowledge.

We are a long way here from modern clinical psychiatry. According to the DSM a patient's doubt becomes hypochondriacal, and therefore pathological, when it persists 'in spite of medical reassurance.' The patient who refuses to yield to medical knowledge finds themselves, by virtue of that refusal, classified as an object of medical knowledge. But can hypochondria really be confined to a clinical diagnosis? Can the ceaseless and contagious doubt that it unleashes be so effectively straitjacketed? Maurice Blanchot once wrote of philosophical scepticism that it is 'invincible,' since the only way it can be defeated is through the deployment of the very forms of rational argumentation that it calls into question. The same might fairly be said of the doubts of those 'fat folder' patients who relentlessly press themselves upon their doctors.

'Hypochondria is the shadow self of medical knowledge,' writes the critic Catherine Belling, 'its always-doubting alter ego.' For Belling this isn't simply because the hypochondriac enjoys discoursing with the confidence of the trained professional, but also because of the doubt that is intrinsic to medicine. We like to think of medicine as omniscient, but when it really comes to define your life, certainties are very promptly replaced by probabilities (a single brusque conversation with someone in a hurry is usually enough to settle matters). A recent study of second opinions across all areas of medicine showed that in 66 percent of cases the diagnosis significantly altered, and in 21 percent of cases, changed entirely. Full agreement between the respective doctors' interpretations occurred only 12 percent of the time. Naturally, misdiagnosis can apply to hypochondria itself.

In the gap that opens between medicine's purportedly complete knowledge of the body and the always-limited insights that it ever truly enjoys, hypochondria enters. Hypochondria, writes Belling, 'is not the patient's illness. It is a condition of knowledge that exceeds medicine's classification of health and disease because the content of hypochondria concerns the very capacity to make that classification in the first place.'

This is what clinical accounts of hypochondria fail to account for. Tony Hancock's joke hinges on the ease with which a person who believed themselves to be suffering from every illness except one would be diagnosed to be suffering from a single illness; and on how, in a neat little irony, the single illness from which they were really suffering would be the very one they were certain that they didn't have. As though hypochondria were the opposite of illness; which, in today's medicalized societies, turns out also to be illness.

In fact as Hancock's joke has it, being diagnosed as 'having' hypochondria means being wrong twice over: not having whatever illness you thought you had, and having the one illness you were certain you didn't have; this agrees with modern clinical definitions of hypochondria, which tend to foreground the erroneousness of hypochondriac fears.

Its inclusion in official diagnostic manuals such as the WHO's IDC-11 (where, like other diagnoses, it includes 'clinical features' and 'developmental presentations') creates the impression that hypochondria, like hypothyroidism, is an illness – a clinical entity whose 'boundaries with other disorders and conditions' can be clearly delineated. Accordingly, hypochondriacs truly are sick – only not in the way they believe. So whatever else it is, a diagnosis of hypochondria is always polemical: a counter-argument in a debate between a patient and a diagnostician with regards to the nature of the patient's problem.

According to contemporary psychiatry, hypochondria is a mental illness 'based on the person's misinterpretation of bodily symptoms.' But if hypochondria is a hermeneutic condition, then I don't think this can be confined to the interpretations, or misinterpretations, of particular problem patients. This is what became clear as I set out to write my serious, scholarly study. Hypochondria gnaws at the edges of the disciplines through which the body becomes an object of knowledge; it thrives in the gaps between the certainty that medicine appears to promise and the uncertainty to which we are always actually confined. In this way it addresses itself to the broader and more uncomfortable truth that, however well-founded, every diagnosis is an act of interpretation.

For all its tenacity, there is something wispy about hypochondria, with its preference for the slight and subtle, its attunement to what might be nothing at all. To be a hypochondriac is to assign the most important role in one's life to something that no one else believes is real, and therefore to embrace a certain tenuousness. Little wonder it is often called 'phantom illness.'

Alone and 'afflicted with hypochondria,' Jean des Esseintes, the protagonist of Joris-Karl Huysmans's *Against Nature*, finds that 'his hand, still firm when it seized a heavy object, trembled when it held a tiny glass.' Likewise, at those times when I could take hold of something weighty – a death, a crisis – I always found my grip to be steady enough. And while I never wished death on anyone, I did come to long for those moments when something else took over, those periods of remission from the everyday when time condensed around something solid and life took on the quality of an event.

I think this is why it was always worst at night: with nothing else to distract it, my mind latched onto vaguer things. Shapes flickered overhead, my ears sang, while thoughts that had been successfully banished during the day passed freely into consciousness. Most crucifying of all was the thought that I had let another day slip by, another day in which, had initiative and resolve not once again been found wanting, I might have done something about it. That whatever was going to happen to me, it would be entirely my fault. No sooner would this thought occur to me than a parade of awful images would dance across my mind's eye.

Friends knew about all of this, knew that I worried about my health, that I was spending a lot of time at the doctor. But I don't think any of them really understood just how much of my mind had been given over to these fears which, even at their peak, I knew might be unfounded. None of this speaks to any failure of empathy; the gap separating our minds was greater than that. In fact, even for me, as I look back today, it is only with a sort of amused contempt that I can look upon that anxious sleeper.

*

'Everyone who is born holds dual citizenship, in the kingdom of the well and in the kingdom of the sick,' writes Susan Sontag at the beginning of *Illness as Metaphor*. 'Although we all prefer to use only the good passport, sooner or later each of us is obliged, at least for a spell, to identify ourselves as citizens of that other place.'

With these metaphors, Sontag is suggesting that there is a clear border separating health and sickness. This is a defining feature of the medicine that has flourished in the liberal economies of the West – where, as Artie Vierkant and Beatrice Adler-Bolton have argued in *Health Communism*, 'health' and 'sickness' are heavily politicized, and policed, terms that determine who does and who does not deserve access to state provisions that are always, and by definition, supposed to be scarce. The Marxist critic David Harvey has gone so far as to argue that sickness under capitalism is defined as the inability to work. This is the reflection that leads Deleuze to hear an expression of hypochondria in Bartleby's enigmatic statement 'I would prefer not to' – words that wreak havoc and disrupt the flow of capital in Melville's famous 'Story of Wall Street.' And so we might say that, a full citizen of neither kingdom, the hypochondriac quietly protests capitalism's ableist demand that the 'healthy' body always be a productive body.

A recent Autoimmune Association survey found that more than 45 percent of patients who go on to be diagnosed with autoimmune diseases have been labelled hypochondriacs in the early stages of their illnesses, while in the United States half of those who go on to be diagnosed with endometriosis – a potentially debilitating condition affecting 10–15 percent of people with wombs – report being initially misdiagnosed with a psychological condition, with physical diagnosis taking on average seven and a half years from the first appearance of symptoms.

This is a recent chapter in a long history of conditions being labelled psychosomatic when their symptoms fall outside the paradigms of current knowledge. In the nineteenth century, for instance, sufferers of multiple sclerosis were often regarded as hysterics, while the neurological symptoms of tertiary syphilis were regarded as a form of moral insanity. It is only very recently (largely due to the sheer extent of long COVID) that the sufferers of post-viral conditions have begun to receive widespread recognition for the physiological basis of their symptoms.

However, we have to acknowledge that here we are also in the territory of the so-called 'contested' diagnoses such as Morgellons disease, a condition with no accepted medical basis, whose self-proclaimed sufferers have formed themselves into online advice and advocacy groups as they aspire to the patienthood that would recognize (and listening to some of them, one is tempted to say alleviate) their suffering. For psychiatry, sufferers of Morgellons are indeed sick, but not in the way they think; in fact they are suffering from a mental illness called 'delusional parasitosis.' Meanwhile in the late nineteenth century, when around one in ten adult men in Britain had syphilis – a disease that could lie dormant for decades and which, at that time, had no test or cure – newspapers and psychiatry manuals began warning of an epidemic of a new disease, responsible for a string of suicides, that was variously called syphilophobia or venereal hypochondriasis.

All of which is to say that hypochondria is never simply the patient's condition. The question of who the hypochondriac is, what's the matter with them, always speaks to the current position of medical knowledge – the ways in which, at any given moment, its categories account for, and do not fully account for, the spectrum of human suffering. Some of those people who currently fall outside of medical categories will eventually come to experience the ambiguous benefits of inclusion; others won't. Hypochondria, therefore, can function like a sort of waiting room, albeit one in which not everyone's name will finally be called.

We would prefer to believe that there is a definite border separating the normal and the pathological because this would make it is possible, at least in theory, to know for certain that one is on the right side of it. If the hypochondriac is rarely a welcome presence, then surely this is partly down to the way they cast light on the unsteady boundary separating health and illness, the fact that it is not fixed once and for all, the way it continues to shift as diseases are discovered, reformulated, reimagined.

We might say, then, that hypochondria serves as a useful, if humbling, reminder of the limits of medicine's knowledge. In which case, the peremptory confinement of the hypochondriac to the ranks of the mentally ill – a patient whose symptoms might be treated, say, with antidepressants or some sessions of CBT (an 'anxietyectomy') – represents a denial of those limits. Moreover, making this judgment would require us to assume a diagnostic omniscience that begins to make the hypochondriac's uncertainty seem like the more credible position. I'm not denigrating medical knowledge, but I am suggesting that by suspending the diagnostic impulse – our claim to know for certain either way – we're able to catch sight of an uncomfortable question that is posed by the hypochondriac. A question that cuts right to the core of all of our relationships, as thinking beings, to our physical bodies: to what extent do we ever *know* that we are healthy?

In recent years clinicians have started to avoid using the word 'hypochondria' in favour of more neutral-sounding terms. Throughout the years during which I was on nodding terms with the clerical staff at my GP's office, 'hypochondria' was not a word I ever heard mentioned, but it was often put to me that I was suffering from an anxiety disorder.

It was around this time that I first read Jean-Paul Sartre's *Being and Nothingness*, with its ennobling descriptions of existential angst. For Sartre, as for Kierkegaard and Heidegger before him, anxiety was not a psychological disorder. It was an existentially rich mood that entailed a hearty acknowledgement of one's own freedom. Thus, a condition of an unenslaved life. More recently, the critic Sianne Ngai has pointed toward anxiety's preeminent position within the West's hierarchy of affects. As a form of anxiety, however, hypochondria appears to have little cultural value; it is, as the critic Elias Canetti writes, in a telling phrase, 'the small change of Angst; it is Angst which for its distraction seeks names and finds them.' Where an existentialist tradition has given us the image of the anxious individual bravely training his eyes on the Nothing, the hypochondriac's gaze is forever being diverted by 'something,' be it a lump or a blemish. 'The hypochondriac,' writes Kierkegaard, is someone who 'is anxious about every insignificant thing.'

In his discussion of 'bad faith,' the ruses and procedures via which people deny their own freedom, Sartre points to how the viewpoint of the hypochondriac is always 'eliminated from the conclusion' of the physician. Labelling someone a hypochondriac means inuring oneself from the possibility of being swayed to their point of view, for the reason that, like the malingering narrator of Ford Madox Ford's *The Good Soldier*, they have ceased to be a reliable narrator of their own experience.

Surely this is the real reason why people who are labelled hypochondriac get so touchy. Not, as the DSM has it, because the word itself is 'pejorative,' a breach of clinical politesse requiring a terminological remedy. But because a doctor who views their patient as a hypochondriac – or as a sufferer of illness anxiety disorder – will disregard their point of view; will eliminate it when coming to form a clinical conclusion.

In *The Invisible Kingdom*, Meghan O'Rourke describes suffering from undiagnosed autoimmune illness, an experience she describes as 'living at the edge of medical knowledge.' She writes, 'In the middle of the night, when I woke in the dark with my heart pounding, what really terrified me was the conviction that … I would never have partners in my search for answers – and treatments. How could I get better if no one thought I was sick?' O'Rourke is pointing to something important, which is the fact that diagnosis starts with conversation. A patient, or a would-be patient, visits their doctor's office having had some out-of-the-ordinary experience – a headache, say, mild but persistent. They attempt to convey this experience. This involves an act of translation. Here is how Virginia Woolf describes the scene:

> let a sufferer try to describe a pain in his head to a doctor and language at once runs dry. There is nothing ready made for him. He is forced to coin words himself, and, taking his pain in one hand, and a lump of pure sound in the other … so to crush them together that a brand new word in the end drops out. Probably it will be something laughable.

Woolf describes this as a poetic task. Perhaps. But it is also rhetorical, a feat of persuasion. The people whom O'Rourke wishes were 'partners in [her] search for answers' are the doctors who are responsible for ordering the scans and tests that will make the body speak; and before this can happen, they need to be won over to the patient's way of seeing things.

So, when Oliver Sacks tells us that the 'patient presents his "story" with a naive immediacy' to a physician who 'listens not just sympathetically but knowledgeably,' I can't help but feel that this is an idealization – not of the physician who knows but of the patient who doesn't. What patient doesn't 'know' these days? My speech was never naive, and if it seemed it, this itself was a performance. Essentially, I was engaged in a kind of lobbying. I knew what I wanted: what test to placate what fear. I also knew that being labelled a hypochondriac, a bad-faith interlocutor, was a threat to all that.

In a desire to economize on my trips to the doctor, I would sometimes seek alternative paths to diagnosis, as on several occasions when I visited the optician because I knew they would use an ophthalmoscope to examine my optic nerve, which, I had learned online, if there was some lesion on my brain, might be enlarged due to the increased pressure inside my skull, a phenomenon called optic neuritis. And on the occasions when I did visit the doctor, I was always very careful to limit what I said, not wishing to appear like one of those knowledgeable patients, a hypochondriac, who turns up requesting a second opinion on a diagnosis that they themselves have made.

A man goes to the doctor, who diagnoses him with hypochondria. 'Oh God,' says the man, 'is it serious?'

Writing about hypochondria forces one to acknowledge a simple truth: that hypochondriacs are funny. If the hypochondriac is so often the butt of the joke, it's surely because of the gap between perception and reality: the way he is forever taking as a matter of life and death what is really nothing at all.

My resort to the masculine pronoun here is not incidental. There is a long comic tradition, beginning with Molière's *Le malade imaginaire*, according to which the hypochondriac is cultured yet ridiculous, middle-class, middle-aged, neurotic, white, and *male*.

Until as recently as the end of the nineteenth century, it was common for medical writers to express the view that hypochondria could only be exhibited in men (with hysteria being reserved for women) while, across the board, nervous ailments were considered to be a form of suffering too refined for people of coarsened working-class or racialized stock. The hypochondriacs we meet with in life are more diverse, and in the clinical literature incidence of hypochondriasis and health anxiety are generally not reported to have any relation to social class or gender identity.

But this is not to say that in the twenty-first century, hypochondria does not intersect with questions of politics and privilege. The privilege, for instance, of living in an industrialized nation, and with free and easy access to medical information. Or under a system of socialized healthcare, such as that of the UK (even as it is torn apart by privatization), as opposed to that of the United States, a country where certain members of the worried well can enjoy limitless choice while window-shopping for ailments at the same time that millions of the un- or under-insured can barely afford a blood test. Anne Boyer points to what she calls her 'reverse hypochondria,' a form of denial, she writes, that was 'reinforced by the rigours of [her] poverty … Everyone knows that in the United States there is no budget for an uninsured mother's illness after the rent and food.' Under capitalism, that is to say, there may be those who lack the resources or the leisure time to be ambiguously unwell.

If hypochondria points toward the limits of medical knowledge, then it is also important to remember that ignorance rarely refers to a plain absence, a neutral gap in what is known. Ignorance, Eve Kosofsky Sedgwick reminds us, is not 'a single Manichaean, aboriginal maw of darkness from which the heroics of human cognition can occasionally wrestle facts.' Instead, she writes, there exist 'a plethora of ignorances, and we may begin to ask questions about the labor, erotics, and economics of their human production and distribution.' According to the philosopher Nancy Tuana, one of the many ways in which ignorance is produced is through the construction of 'epistemically disadvantaged identities,' while Miranda Fricker describes the 'epistemic injustice' faced by the 'hermeneutically marginalized.' Which is to say that identifying the hypochondriac is always a political task, encoded by histories that have famously been kinder to certain groups than to others.

According to Naomi Klein, 'women's legitimate complaints are too often discounted, dismissed, or disbelieved as hypochondria.' The effects of this are very real. Medical credibility has repeatedly been shown to have an enormous impact on the quality of health outcomes, and to fluctuate according to class, gender, and race.

Women are seven times more likely to be misdiagnosed and discharged in the middle of a heart attack, while women with chronic pain conditions are more likely than men to be misdiagnosed with, and treated for, mental health conditions. Meanwhile, as Klein explains, these 'failures and abandonments by conventional medicine are vastly more severe for Black and Indigenous women, who are consistently treated as unreliable narrators of their own bodies.' According to multiple studies Black patients are systematically undertreated for pain, with the wisdoms of nineteenth-century race science – that Black people have less sensitive nerve endings or 'thicker skin' – having maintained their hold over the majority-white medical imagination (according to a 2016 study, the latter claim is believed by nearly half of all white first-year medical students in the United States). In the UK, Black women are half as likely to be diagnosed with endometriosis as white women, while in the US and UK mortality rates in childbirth among Black women are respectively three and four times higher than among white women.

The production of medical ignorance is not simply a case of who is and who is not believed. Endometriosis affects only those with wombs. When it comes to autoimmune disorders, 80 percent of sufferers are women; and in the case of a specific autoimmune disorder, lupus, incidence among Black and Hispanic women is around three times greater than among non-Hispanic white women. All these conditions are under-researched. There is a circular logic at work: research into diseases that disproportionately affect more marginalized groups tends to be underfunded, and this in turn increases the likelihood that the narratives of people suffering from these conditions will fall outside the current paradigms of medical knowledge, meaning they are more likely to present in clinical settings as 'difficult' patients.

This is the context in which nearly half of the people who, like O'Rourke, are eventually diagnosed as having an auto-immune disorder are initially labelled hypochondriac. As Tuana writes, in instances such as these, 'it is not simply facts, events, practices, or technologies that are rendered not known, but individuals and groups who are rendered "not knowers."'

In popular imagination, the hypochondriac is a familiar character: zany and neurotic, a notorious buttonholer who enjoys enumerating his symptoms and nursing his fictitious ailments. However, the comic trope of the imaginary invalid may obscure the extent to which, in reality, medical credibility – the question of who is and isn't deemed a reliable narrator of their own body – and the health outcomes this produces tend to follow another, equally familiar pattern.

*

O'Rourke's fears are vividly realized in a posthumously published letter by Lisa Steen, a doctor who at the time of writing it was suffering from kidney cancer with multiple bone metastases, with only a few weeks to live. Steen describes having her concerns dismissed by several of her medical colleagues, at which point she was consigned to 'two years wandering in the wilderness of the medically unexplained.' Throughout this time, she was experiencing visual impairments as well as 'fatigue, palpitations, cramps in my hands and feet, subtle cognitive impairments, difficulty finding words, memory problems, difficulty coping at work' – nebulous symptoms that were disregarded as stress, or as side effects of the antidepressant medications she was prescribed to manage her 'anxiety.' After she died, her husband told a newspaper, 'They didn't seem to be taking her too seriously, particularly because she had been diagnosed with health anxiety, she was being looked at as a hypochondriac.'

Certain that what Steen was suffering from was a psychological ailment, her doctors were unable to sufficiently investigate other possible causes of her symptoms. Stories like this used to make my heart stop. This is what every hypochondriac fears; it is the point at which the joke becomes serious. Being designated a hypochondriac by the person capable of administering – and withholding – referrals, tests, and scans can feel like, and let's state it plainly, might be, a matter of life and death.

*

Perhaps, then, there is another reason why hypochondria is often referred to as 'phantom illness.' After all, in the fullness of time it is always possible that *hypochondria* will be revealed to be the illness from which one was not really suffering. This is the sting in the tail of a joke, told by Slavoj Žižek, in which a doctor says to his patient: 'First the good news. We established you are definitely not a hypochondriac.' Brian Dillon writes that hypochondria 'makes dupes of us all, because life, or rather death, will have the last laugh.' Hypochondria is a sort of comedy of errors, a joke in which the punchline is always the same – until it isn't, since, as every hypochondriac knows, sooner or later they are fated to be correct, heralding that terrible and delectable moment of vindication: I told you I was ill.

One would like to imagine that these words, the famous epitaph of Tony Hancock's friend and collaborator Spike Milligan, constitute something of a moral victory over hypochondria, perhaps even mortality, or maybe just one's friends. I myself have not always been immune to this proleptic fantasy. Back in my early twenties I would play the scene over and over in my imagination, enlisting a revolving cast of incredulous confidants and exercising full directorial control (EXT. WINTER. A COLD WIND BLOWS).

And even all those years later, now approaching my mid-thirties, as I sat down to write my serious, scholarly study of hypochondria, I found myself imagining the news articles that might be written were it to be revealed, after the book had gone to press (but let's say, just in time for publication), that my fears had in fact been right all along. That in the years during which I'd been calmly reading about the history of imaginary illness a very real disease, no longer curable, had slowly been taking hold. And thinking about this one night I was surprised to experience the resurgence of my old fears, fears that I had not experienced for years and which I quickly put to rest by vowing, if this were to happen, that I would ask my publisher to issue an erratum slip whose laconic correction ('He wasn't really a hypochondriac') would be sure to make my book a surprise commercial success.

Of course I knew the pleasures of this fantasy would in reality be thin. The nothing to which the hypochondriac pledges their life could always turn out to be something, or maybe not, and either way it is hypochondria that is guaranteed to have the last laugh.

Perhaps we ought to simply say that one can never be quite certain of where one stands with hypochondria: it is a condition that is all-consuming yet vanishingly insubstantial, genuinely horrible yet difficult to take seriously. Two faced, like the respectively smiling and frowning faces of comedy and tragedy. That 'strangest spectre,' Charlotte Brontë called it, thus speaking to a phenomenon at once incessant and airy. Maybe this is why, the more I read about hypochondria back in 2020, the less I found myself confidently able to describe it – as though, for all my scholarly aspirations, I was chasing after nothing, grasping at something whose very nature it was to recede from view.

DISAPPEARANCES

For millennia, hypochondria has addressed itself to the relationship between mind and body. With its continual displacements and transformations, hypochondria has been less a stable diagnosis than a question that refuses to go away.

From *hypo-*, meaning below, and *-chondrium*, referring to the cartilage of the ribs. At first *hypochondria* (plural) was an anatomical term referring to two areas of the upper abdomen that sit beneath the costal cartilage on either of the epigastrium, and which contain the liver, spleen, and gallbladder. The first recorded use of the word appears to have been in the (variously authored) writings attributed to Hippocrates of Kos, traditionally considered to be the founder of Western medicine.

Hippocratic medicine aimed at the preservation of health through the correct balance of the humours – four vital substances that were related to the four elements, the four seasons, the four times of day, the four phases of life. Each humour had a set of functions: blood was the source of vitality; choler necessary for digestion; phlegm cooled and lubricated; while black bile or melancholy, produced by the hypochondrium, was the source of pigmentation. The fluctuations of the humours determined states of health and sickness: illness ensued when one humour came to dominate over the others, with the state of torpor, fear, and sadness that was called melancholy being among the consequences of an overactive hypochondrium.

Hippocrates refers to the hypochondrium several times in his collected writings, for instance in the case of a man who, having dined and drunk too heartily, finds himself suffering with vomiting, fever, and 'pain in the right hypochondrium.' By the fourth day the pain has spread all over his body, and on the tenth things have taken a further turn for the worse: 'Legs painful; general exacerbation; wandering.' For the eleventh day, a single word: 'Death.'

It seems to have been some centuries later, in the writings of the second century CE physician Galen of Pergamon, that hypochondria – *morbus hypochondriacus* – was first named as a specific illness. Hypochondria was a subspecies of melancholy, one that in comparison to its kindred plaints retained a particularly close connection to the abdominal region from which it hailed.

In the seventh century, for instance, Paulus of Aegina delineated three forms of melancholia: that of the whole body, that of the brain, and lastly wind melancholia – otherwise called *melancholia flatuosa* or *melancholia hypochondriaca*. A millennium later, Robert Burton would reprise this tripartite distinction, dedicating several long passages of his *Anatomy* to enumerating the symptoms of 'hypochondriacal or flatuous melancholy.'

This etiological theory created a link between hypochondria and flatulence that would prove surprisingly tenacious, remaining unchallenged until the eighteenth century and still a fixture of clinical descriptions well into the Victorian era. In the literature of the period, ideas about digestion merged with another received notion about hypochondria, that it bore some special relationship to intellectual activity. As late as 1807, Thomas Trotter could write in his influential *View of the Nervous Temperament* of the 'highly sensible bowels' of those engaged in intellectual activities. 'Hence,' he explained, 'the numerous instances of dyspepsia, hypochondriasis and melancholia, in the literary character.'

In the 'health diary' that Charles Darwin kept for the five years following his experiments with hydrotherapy in the spring of 1849, which forms a kind of archive of his body, Darwin marshalled his naturalist's sensibility to the task of recording the eruptions of his bowels. Flatulence, often abbreviated to 'flat' or 'ft,' appears to have been experienced frequently and in 'fits' that he diligently categorized as 'slightest,' 'very slight,' 'slight,' and 'almost,' all the way to 'considerable,' 'baddish,' 'rather bad,' 'bad,' 'very bad,' and 'excessive.'

With his health diary, Darwin was bringing a little scientific rigour to a practice that, throughout the eighteenth and nineteenth centuries, became a common pastime for men of letters, who in their diaries and correspondence often took to chronicling the state of their bowels. In his letters Thomas Carlyle complains about 'all [his] dyspepsias, and nervousness and hypochondriasis.' He was 'dying by inches,' he told his brother in 1823 (he died more than half a century later, in 1881). Samuel Beckett is drawing on this august tradition when in *Molloy* he has his dishevelled hero, wrapped up for warmth in copies of the *Times Literary Supplement*, making a similar tally:

> Three hundred and fifteen farts in nineteen hours, or an average of over sixteen farts an hour. After all it's not excessive. Four farts every fifteen minutes. It's nothing. Not even one fart every four minutes. It's unbelievable. Damn it, I hardly fart at all, I should never have mentioned it. Extraordinary how mathematics help you to know yourself.

*

In addition to melancholy, hypochondria was often associated with another ancient condition. Hysteria, as is well known, was generally regarded as a female disorder caused by an errant womb. However, the symptoms of hysteria (spasms, pains, paralysis, psychic distress) were hardly exclusive to women, and so, beginning in the seventeenth century, hypochondria was increasingly proposed as a male counterpart.

Thomas Sydenham, often called the English Hippocrates, claimed that hypochondria 'is as like hysteria as one egg is to another.' In the centuries that followed, this became a common view. In his 1765 *Observations on the Nature, Causes, and Cure of Those Disorders which Have Been Commonly Called Nervous, Hypochondriac, Or Hysteric*, for instance, the Edinburgh doctor Robert Whytt argued that these two labels named male and female versions of a single disease, and that if hysterical symptoms were 'often much more sudden and violent,' then this was 'only a consequence of the more delicate frame, sedentary life, and particular condition of the womb in women.' Thus, beginning in the eighteenth century, hypochondria and hysteria become male and female versions of one disease, a sort of 'his' and 'hers.'

That said, this belief was far from universally accepted. Sydenham's contemporary Thomas Willis regarded any similarities between the conditions as superficial, and, a century later, William Cullen, the most important doctor of his generation, would go so far as to call hypochondria 'exactly opposite' to hysteria. The two conditions were as closely related, he said, as black is to white. Also of note here were other disorders, such as 'the vapours' or 'the spleen,' which were sometimes held to be synonymous with hypochondria, and/or hysteria, and were at other times held to be entirely separate disorders, with symptomatologies and treatment pathways of their own, which a skilled physician could discern via differential diagnosis.

Such debates were mainly of interest to those theoretical writers addressing a medical audience. When it came to books intended for a more general readership distinctions tended to be elided, as can be seen in the capacious subtitle of George Cheyne's spectacularly popular 1735 book *The English Malady: or, A treatise of nervous diseases of all kinds, as spleen, vapours, lowness of spirits, hypochondriacal, and hysterical distempers, &c.* There seems to have been a market logic at play here: by presenting such conditions under a single banner, while insuring against any terminological innovations with a prudent etcetera, Cheyne's book, like many others, could address itself to the widest possible audience.

Whatever view one took, however, it is clear that the symptoms of hysteria and hypochondria developed according to gendered stereotypes in which the body is coded female and the mind male. This became even more apparent throughout the nineteenth century, aided by the development of photography and a nascent science of psychiatry that was based on the observation and classification of positive symptoms. The hysteric was renowned for her paroxysms and convulsions; she was liable to swoon. Her performance drew on an almost infinite repertoire of visible bodily gestures – tics, fits, spasms, and seizures – and yet, most strangely and most touchingly of all, the hysteric herself was said to exist in a state of *belle indifference*; that is, to be blissfully innocent as to the existence of her condition (until the arrival of the male analyst).

What could be further from hypochondria, as it came to be understood? Hypochondria, a condition where in the absence of observable symptoms the sufferer is obsessed with the idea there is something wrong with him. As the critic Steven Connor puts it, while hysteria became the condition that was all symptoms with no interpretation, hypochondria became all interpretation and no symptoms. An intellectual condition, let's call it. Or better still, the intellectual's condition, the never entirely awful outcome of a mind that was working too hard, that couldn't help but pay attention to every inch of the body in which it resided.

Needless to say, hypochondria, which by the end of the nineteenth century was generally deemed to be 'all in the head,' did not produce any significant iconography. How could it? This was in dramatic contrast to the hysteric, whose vivid symptoms could be observed, recorded, and documented – as in the photographs from Jean-Martin Charcot's Salpêtrière, in which we can witness the manifold avatars of hysterical sickness. In his famous Tuesday Lessons, Charcot would have female hysterics theatrically demonstrate their symptoms for the edification and entertainment of Europe's medical elite, a scene, perhaps a primal scene, famously captured by André Brouillet's *A Clinical Lesson at the Salpêtrière*, which shows Charcot lecturing before an assembly of men with his swooning patient, Marie Wittman, her arms behind her like two twisted ropes. Freud obtained a lithograph of the painting in 1889 and hung it in his consulting room. When he moved to London, in 1938, driven out of Vienna by the Nazis, he had it hung over his analytic couch, where it remains to this day, enjoyed by visitors to what is now the Freud Museum, taken away on postcards that cost a pound.

If, by comparison, the hypochondriac has been a fairly neglected figure, then he has at least been spared the many indignities that come with fame. For centuries the hypochondriac, when not being ignored, has been a figure of affectionate contempt. He raises eyebrows but rarely stirs more violent thoughts. It has never occurred to anyone to confine him. One simply teases him a little, and if that proves ineffective, avoids him.

In a paradoxical sort of way, then, hypochondria can be a culturally normalizing script. At times throughout history, it has afforded, to a certain type of privileged male, a degree of self-indulgence and eccentricity rarely granted to women. In Wilkie Collins's *The Woman in White* Frederick Fairlie indulges his hypochondriac foibles from the safety of his bedroom, where he remains largely untouched by the novel's plot; meanwhile his niece Anne is placed in an asylum as part of an economic scheme, her attempts to resist this treated as further evidence of her insanity. Whether calculating or insane, and whether to society or to herself, a woman's madness has always been treated as somehow more threatening than a man's.

When lockdown set in, I had to make do without the British Library and the books I needed for my research. Perhaps this was fortuitous; when the narrator of Jerome K. Jerome's Three Men in a Boat visits the British Library, he ends up diagnosing himself with nearly every disease in the medical dictionary: 'I had walked into that reading-room a happy, healthy man. I crawled out a decrepit wreck.'

For centuries medical authorities have warned about the dangers of excessive reading. This view seems to have originated in *Problems*, a text that was long believed to have been authored by Aristotle (though which in reality was compiled by different authors, in the spirit of his philosophy, over the course of several centuries). 'Why is it,' the pseudo-Aristotelean text asks, 'that all men who have become outstanding in philosophy, statesmanship, poetry or the arts are melancholic'? The author goes on to name Empedocles, Socrates, and Plato as only a few of the eminent men who have suffered from an excess of the black bile.

In the second century CE, this connection between learning and melancholy was maintained by the physician Rufus of Ephesus, and later by Cicero. In the fifteenth century the Italian priest and Neoplatonist scholar Marsilio Ficino would approvingly cite *Problems*, thus reinventing the melancholic genius as a figure of the Renaissance. Ficino argued that the most dedicated students and scholars tended to fall under the influence of Saturn (he himself was born under that star), with this fact accounting for both the highs and the lows of intellectual endeavour.

With Ficino, melancholia became a coveted label among members of the Florentine Neoplatonist elite, and soon after, beyond. Gutenberg's new printing press meant that these ideas could permeate through Europe at unprecedented speed, spreading first to Germany, and then to Britain. As the historian Matthew Bell tells us in his book *Melancholia: The Western Malady*, by the time Shakespeare sat down to write *Hamlet* at the end of the sixteenth century, Ficino's notion of melancholy genius had become embedded in English courtly life.

Throughout the European Renaissance, countless paintings and engravings would depict the melancholic, typically seen alone in his study, flanked by his books. The most famous example is Albrecht Dürer's *Melencolia I*, in which the figure of Melancholy is surrounded by discarded tools: hourglass, hammer, scales, plane, and saw – implements which, for all their earthly utility, fail to get the measure of the celestial sphere, and therefore speak to a craving for knowledge that can only but go unsatisfied.

The following century, an etched frontispiece to Burton's *Anatomy of Melancholy* depicts the different types of melancholic: Solitudo, Inamorato, Superstitiosus, Maniacus, and Hypochondriacus. The latter is represented as an aged gentleman, fur-clad though indoors. Scattered around him is an extensive pharmacopeia of nostrums, while overhead the symbol ♄ informs us that he has fallen under the sign of Saturn. An accompanying verse outlining 'The Argument of the Frontispiece' reads:

Hypochondriacus leans on his arm,
Winde in his side doth him much harm,
And troubles him full sore, God knows,
Much pain he hath and man, woes.
About him pots and glasses lie,
Newly brought from's Apothecary.
This Saturn's aspects signifie,
You see them portraid in the skie.

According to Burton, above all it was a 'sedentary, solitary life' and 'overmuch learning' that all but condemned the scholar to melancholy, while hypochondria named a form of melancholy whose sufferers were distinguished for making frequent visits to the apothecarist and for their extravagant bodily delusions, such as, most famously, the belief that it had been turned into earthenware or glass.

With the waning authority of humoral medicine in the seventeenth and eighteenth centuries, melancholy increasingly went by the name of hypochondria, now recast as a disease of the nervous system, a network of vanishingly slight vessels that suffused the body with animal spirits.

The connection with learning was easy to absorb into this new etiology. Thomas Sydenham wrote of 'such male subjects as lead a sedentary or studious life, and grow pale over their books and papers.' In his essay 'Of the Complaints of Men of Learning' Vicesimus Knox suggested that 'that lowness of spirits which a sedentary life, and an unremitted attention produce, may give rise to complaints founded only in an hypochondriac imagination.' Robert Whytt popularized the view that nervous diseases were primarily caused by heightened sensibility. It was hardly surprising, then, that 'the studious' were the demographic who were 'most subject to hypochondriac disorders.' With the help of medical works like Whytt's, the eighteenth century erected a cult of sensibility in which nervous ailments like hypochondria were a painful, if not entirely unwelcome, over-development of the capacity to feel.

It was during a summer break from Pembroke College, Oxford, that Samuel Johnson succumbed to what, years later, his younger friend James Boswell would call 'an horrible hypo-chondria ... with a dejection, gloom, and despair, which made existence misery.' In the throes of an attack, Johnson feared that he would lose touch with reality, and in this confused state, his sensorium became so disordered that he could no longer distinguish the time on the town clock. The return of his hypochondria became Johnson's worst fear. A recursive and tautological fear, therefore: an anxiety whose main object was anxiety.

The physician Robert James probably had his learned friend in mind when he wrote in his *Medicinal Dictionary* (to which Johnson contributed) that hypochondria was 'very common among the Literati,' while in *An Essay on Diseases Incidental to Literary and Sedentary Persons*, the celebrated Swiss physician Samuel-Auguste Tissot agreed.

Boswell would consult Tissot in the midst of his own nervous crisis while studying in Holland. Later, he wrote: 'We Hypochondriacks … console ourselves in the hour of gloomy distress, by thinking that our suffering marks our superiority.' Johnson reproached his friend for his youthful tendency to equate hypochondria with intellect. By the end of the eighteenth century, hypochondria had become modish, such that anyone wishing to convey an air of erudition or sensitivity could do worse than to affect a certain gloominess. Writing in his 1790 book *Essays on Fashionable Diseases*, James Makittrick Adair addressed Robert Whytt's book about hypochondria: 'Before the publication of this book, people of fashion had not the least idea that they had nerves.' Now anyone who was anyone (or who wished to be someone) was feigning nervousness. In the view of a growing number of doctors like Adair, the vast literature about nervous illness was not simply describing hypochondria – it was transmitting it.

As a young teacher, Charlotte Brontë fell prey to 'Hypochondria – A most dreadful doom.' Years later, in a letter that she wrote to her friend and former employer while she was at work on Jane Eyre, Brontë describes the 'preternatural horror which seemed to clothe existence and Nature – and which made life a continual waking Nightmare.' Hypochondria, she explains, is a state of agonizing receptivity, in which the 'morbid Nerves can know neither peace nor enjoyment – whatever touches – pierces them – sensation for them is all suffering.'

From the late eighteenth century on, hypochondria was often seen as a form of nervous susceptibility, a painfully heightened perception. Edgar Allan Poe writes of Roderick Usher, the sickly aristocrat whose physical fate is bound, in some obscure way, to that of the crumbling house in which he lives:

> He suffered much from a morbid acuteness of the senses; the most insipid food was alone endurable; he could wear only garments of certain texture; the odors of all flowers were oppressive; his eyes were tortured by even a faint light; and there were but peculiar sounds, and these from stringed instruments, that did not inspire him with horror.

In Huysmans's *Against Nature*, des Esseintes seems to be suffering from a similar affliction. Self-cure and symptom converge as he sets about controlling every aspect of his environment. His aim is to ensure that his senses are only greeted by the most salutary phenomena, a plan that, like every totalizing scheme, ends up exacerbating the malaise that it's intended to ameliorate.

Likewise, Brontë insists that the pain caused by hypochondria is 'far worse than that of a man with healthy nerves buried for the same length of time in a subterranean dungeon.' In describing her own experience, Brontë equates hypochondria with suffering plain and simple. But when it comes to be reimagined in her fiction, the condition is never without its ambiguous privileges. Though doubtlessly of a gloomy cast, hypochondriacs, as Brontë imagines them through her fiction, possess a unique kind of insight.

Based on Brontë's years as a teacher in Belgium, *Villette* is bathed in a sad, grey ambience. The narrator, Lucy Snowe, is by turns withdrawn and alert – estranged from her surroundings and from her own emotions, yet always ready to savage an unsuspecting (and sometimes undeserving) interlocutor with a cruel remark. The reason for these vicissitudes of personality appears to lie in the duplicitous condition to which she has been consigned, a condition that waxes and wanes according to an opaque agenda of its own but that, crucially, insists on conspiring with its sufferer:

> Hypochondria has that wont, to rise in the midst of thousands – dark as Doom, pale as Malady, and well-nigh strong as Death. Her comrade and victim thinks to be happy one moment – 'Not so,' says she; 'I come.' And she freezes the blood in his heart, and beclouds the light in his eye.

Regarding any comradely element of her own hypochondria, Brontë is silent. But other writers have been more candid. Kierkegaard cherished his 'holy hypochondria.' For Kafka hypochondria was unavoidable, the natural course for someone whose 'whole being is directed toward literature'; and while he frequently complained about it, he also feared that any cessation of his anxiety could only come 'at the expense of [his] writing.'

'His eye and his sense of smell never missed the slightest thing,' writes Céleste Albaret, erstwhile maid to Marcel Proust. Albaret describes the bizarre rigmarole of his care: the walls sound-proofed with cork; the bottles of Evian mineral water that were continually replaced even though no drop of liquid, save for cups of thick Corcellet coffee, ever passed Proust's lips. For Albaret this sensitivity was all part of Proust's literary genius, and in her fond yet chilling descriptions she comes close to endowing him with psychical powers.

But it is with Thomas Mann's *The Magic Mountain* that we find the fullest expression of hypochondria's covert privileges. In Mann's novel illness is a kind of sentimental education. The uncultivated bourgeois Hans Castorp visits the mountaintop sanatorium to see his cousin. He plans to stay for three weeks but after developing a mild fever goes on to spend seven years reading and reclining – and only occasionally coughing – in this elevated setting nestled between the kingdoms of the sick and of the well.

This ambivalence is captured by an artistic tradition that seems to have been popularized by Ficino, in which melancholy was represented via the respectively smiling and frowning faces of Democritus and Heraclitus, known as 'the laughing philosopher' and 'the weeping philosopher' because of their diverging responses to the folly of the world. Ficino adorned his study with a painting of the two philosophers, pictured on either side of a world globe. Taken together, their contrasting faces express the affective range of a duplicitous condition that, according to most medical authorities, could produce delight as well as dejection.

*

It's worth returning to Burton's *Anatomy of Melancholy*. Surely, it is one of the strangest books ever written. Burton wrote openly about his own melancholy, which he attributed to the rigours of scholarly life; and yet he also expressed the hope that researching and writing the *Anatomy* might relieve him of his condition. Indeed, while he had been known to 'lament with Heraclitus,' Burton threw his lot in with the laughing philosopher, publishing his book under the pseudonym 'Democritus Junior.'

Burton seems to have been particularly struck by a story, told by Hippocrates, about how the doctor came upon Democritus dissecting animal corpses in a fruitless search for the anatomical 'cause of madness and melancholy.' Substituting scalpel for pen, Burton also sought to 'anatomize and cut up' each aspect of this disease, a disease whose symptoms, he wrote, 'are irregular, obscure, various, so infinite, Proteus himself is not so diverse, you may as well make the moon a new coat, as a true character of a melancholy man.' If this was true of anyone wishing to understand a single melancholic, then where did this leave the scholar wishing the elucidate the nature of melancholy as such? The first edition of the *Anatomy* was published in 1621. Over the next twenty years Burton revised, which invariably meant expanded, the *Anatomy* five times. This culminated in a vast posthumously published 1651 edition. When it was completed (if that is the word) shortly before Burton's death in 1640, its pages counted more than half again those of the original.

'Hypochondriacal or flatuous melancholy,' Burton explains, 'is in my judgment the most grievous and frequent' form of melancholy. Here are some of the symptoms its sufferers endure:

Their ears sing now and then, vertigo and giddiness come by fits, turbulent dreams, dryness, leanness, apt they are to sweat upon all occasions ... Many of them are high-coloured especially after meals ... sometimes their shoulders and shoulder blades ache, there is a leaping all over their bodies, sudden trembling, a palpitation of the heart ... short breath, hard wind, strong pulse, swooning.

Despite this long list of physical symptoms, Burton writes of hypochondriacal melancholy that 'most commonly fear, grief, and some sudden commotion, or perturbation of the mind, begin it.' During the early-modern period, the brain had not acquired dominance over the other organs, and the viscera were sometimes regarded to be the seat of the imagination. Writing around the same time as Burton, Jan Baptist van Helmont, the influential chemist, argued that the soul resided in the stomach and spleen ('If a gun sends forth a noise unexpectedly,' van Helmont observed not unreasonably, one 'feels the token of fear in the mouth of his stomach'). Diseases of the soul occurred whenever these organs fell under the sway of an 'idea morbosa,' which meant that according to the medical wisdom of the time, hypochondria could be imaginary without, for this reason, being unreal: it began with the influence of morbid ideas, but those ideas soon became transformed into material realities.

If ideas alone could make a person sick, then where did this leave the reader of a vast tract on melancholy? Wasn't there the risk that this person would come away from it the worse? Burton was aware of the threat:

one caution let me give by the way to my … reader, who is actually melancholy, that he read not the symptoms or prognostics in this following tract, lest by applying that which he reads to himself, aggravating, appropriating things generally spoken, to his own person (as melancholy men for the most part do) he trouble or hurt himself, and get in conclusion more harm than good.

This was not the last time that hypochondriacs would be warned to avoid reading lists of medical symptoms. Hypochondria, wrote Kant one hundred and fifty years later, can 'be called fictitious disease, in which the patient finds in himself symptoms of every disease he reads about in books.'

In the nineteenth century, this would become standard medical wisdom. In Britain, successive Education Acts meant that between 1800 and 1900 illiteracy fell from around 50 percent to 3 percent. As this took place, medical authorities began to worry about the effect this would have on the public, in particular on women, whose nerves were finer and more delicate. This period also saw an explosion of popular medical books that catered to, and perhaps created, an increasingly health-conscious population. As medical knowledge ceased to be the preserve of physicians, members of that profession began to worry about the consequences, with one physician decrying the spread of 'pernicious books of "popular medicine," innumerable copies of which are in circulation all over the world.' There is, he wrote, 'no doubt that the reading of this kind of literature has often resulted in an attack of hypochondriasis.'

It was now, as ever greater swathes of the population were being transformed into readers, that hypochondria began to lose its connection with the abdomen, settling into its current meaning: hypochondria as a hermeneutic condition in which (as the DSM puts it) one suffers not from physical symptoms themselves but the way one 'interprets them.' Where a glance at the Renaissance literature reveals that hypochondriacs once suffered from colourful delusions – the baker who believed he was made of butter and so refused to go near the bread ovens; the man who, believing himself to be a nightingale, sang all night long – in our age of widespread medical literacy, hypo-chondriacal fantasies tend to be grounded in stolid medical possibilities. Rarely fanciful, they are all too plausible.

The Victorian age saw the emergence of a vast medical litera-ture, a mass of information, advice, and opinion which, in the twenty-first century, finds its apotheosis in the internet. The internet has put medical information ever at our fingertips, and has turned the least scholarly of us into readers. And so it should perhaps come as little surprise that, since the early 2000s, medical writers have been warning about a new scourge, 'cyberchondria.' (For those who fear they might be suffering from this condition: '5 Ways to Tell if You Have Cyberchondria' [*Psychology Today*]; '15 Signs You're a Cyberchondriac' [*Yahoo*].)

An anonymous reviewer for *The Lancet* perhaps foresaw this in 1855 when he decried the way that popular medical books were 'incessantly vomited forth by the press.' 'It is clear,' the reviewer writes, 'that works of this character are intended for hypochondriacal reading … It would be a waste of time to peruse them with the hope of deriving any useful information.'

Late in the eighteenth century, William Cullen gave what might be the first description of modern hypochondria: 'As it is the nature of men to indulge every present emotion, so the hypochondriac cherishes his fears, and attentive to every feeling, finds in trifles, light as air, a strong confirmation of his apprehensions.' In this psychologically rich description, it is a particular attitude that takes precedence, with any physical element being the result of the hypochondriac's heightened attention: hypochondria concerned the body, but increasingly it belonged to the mind. Across the Victorian era, views like these came to predominate. In contrast to Burton's sharp belchings and fulsome crudities, hypochondria became an airy phenomenon in which mental states pulled free from their grounding in bodily realities. While eighteenth-century medical books still talk about the alimentary canal, by 1897 it is possible for a popular textbook to note, 'In hypochondriasis the patient suffers from a purely mental malady.'

It is now, as it is absorbed into the new category of the diseases of the mind, that hypochondria first starts to acquire pejorative connotations. In hypochondria 'the mind is affected as much as and possibly more than the body,' wrote the French physician Joseph Lieutaud – 'hence the term hypochondriac has become almost an offensive name avoided by physicians who aim to please.' With no physical etiology, hypochondria becomes at best a sign of moral or emotional laxity, and at worst a form of imposture or malingering.

Despite all this, compared with hysteria, hypochondria was also stubbornly physical. By the turn of the twentieth century, hysteria had come to be understood by Freud's nascent psychoanalytic science as a conversion neurosis, the bodily expression of some psychic conflict. Psychoanalysis was a form of translation: in conversation with her analyst, the hysteric would eventually come to understand the psychological struggle underlying her physical condition.

When it came to hypochondria, opinion was split as to the relationship between its manifest and latent content. Freud's early colleague Alfred Adler described hypochondria as a defence neurosis 'suitable to protect those afflicted with defeats in life.' Conversely, Freud believed that hypochondria was an 'actual' neurosis – a physiological ailment whose psychological aspect was secondary. Basically it was a bodily disease, and so, in its crude literalism, it was of limited analytic interest. In contrast to the confident claims that were often made on behalf of hysterics, it was difficult to say what the hypochondriac 'really' fears. What the hypochondriac fears *may* be the conscious recognition of an unconscious desire. Or it may, in the end, be simply illness.

Hypochondria posed a problem for a psychiatry that was increasingly based on the observation of positive symptoms. At the same time, new technologies revealed the physiological basis of conditions such as anemia and endocrine disorders, whose sufferers might once have been dismissed as hypochondriac to have a physical basis. Though it continued to appear in medical textbooks, its symptomatology generally a hybrid of modern and early-modern wisdom, by the end of the nineteenth century hypochondria had become a minor topic within medical discourse. As the historian Susan Baur has suggested, lacking the clear outlines of a noun, it started to become an adjective ('hypochondriac behaviour') confined to descriptions of other, more definite illnesses.

At the dawn of the twentieth century, hypochondria tended to oscillate between mind and body, between being an illness in its own right and being merely an obsession with illness where none in fact existed.

In 1539 Andreas Vesalius, a professor of surgery and anatomy at the University of Padua, was granted access to the corpses of those who had been executed by the Venetian state and allowed to take them to his laboratory. This was a rare privilege at a time when the dissection of human corpses was subject to a strict taboo.

Vesalius would go on to publish his findings in 1543, the same year that Copernicus published *On the Revolutions of the Celestial Spheres*. Lavishly illustrated in the studio of Titian, *On the Fabric of the Human Body in Seven Books* charted the inner universe of man's body; it overturned centuries of medical doctrine in a way that was no less revolutionary than the thesis of heliocentrism put forward by Copernicus.

Vesalius's findings dealt a blow to the theory of the four humours that, for nearly two thousand years, had defined Western medicine. Soon after publication, the anatomist proceeded to launch a series of extraordinary attacks against his medical forebears, especially Galen, who he claimed had never opened a human corpse and could not even be trusted as a reliable cartographer of the bodies of the apes he dissected instead.

Vesalius's intervention did not spell the immediate end of humoral ideas, but it was the first in a series of developments that sent them into a long decline. A few years later, when the English physician William Harvey published his findings regarding the circulation of blood, he would find little evidence to support the central role that had been assigned to the balance of the other humours, in particular that darkest, most elusive and troublesome fluid.

If black bile was nowhere to be found, what did all this mean for the state of mental and physical unrest called melancholia? As the historian Janet Oppenheim writes, across the seventeenth century, as humoral doctrine was increasingly marginalized by discoveries from the emerging discipline of anatomy, hypochondria gradually began to displace melancholy 'as the generic term for disorders involving low spirits, apprehensiveness, diffuse physical malaise, languor, irritability, and even pain.'

Along with hysteria, hypochondria enabled Enlightenment physicians to elaborate a new type of functional disease that did not arise in any specific organ. The two most important physicians of the seventeenth century, Thomas Willis and Thomas Sydenham, did not completely reject the involvement of the spleen in the etiology of hypochondria. Both, however, had come to view it as a condition of the nervous system. By the end of the eighteenth century, William Cullen could write in his treatise *First Lines of the Practice of Physic* that he 'propose[d] to comprehend, under the title of NEUROSES ... the hysteric or hypochondriacal disorders,' as well as 'all those [others] which do not depend upon a topical affection of the organs, but upon a more general affection of the nervous system.'

Of course, hypochondria was itself deeply entangled in the humoral ideas of Hippocrates and Galen, and so, even in writers like Cullen we see repeated references to the alimentary canal. As an attempt at modernization, hypochondria was in this sense something of a fudge. It was a rickety bridge between the abdomen and the imagination, body and mind, old ideas and newer ones. In years to come, this would increasingly become clear, leading to repeated attempts to reinvent the condition or else to banish it entirely from medical textbooks.

*

Readers of modern psychiatric manuals will notice that hypo-chondria is typically referred to as hypochondriasis. In truth there is no difference between the two terms. The suffix '-sis' – commonly used in medicine to form nouns out of processes or ongoing conditions (tuberculosis, psoriasis) – was added to hypochondria in the second half of the eighteenth century, an early and relatively low-key attempt to reinvent for modern medicine an ancient condition that, it was increasingly under-stood, had little to do with rib cartilage.

Other, more decisive attempts at terminological revolution were to follow. Cullen's 'neurosis' was especially notable, but if you go looking, nineteenth-century medical books are full of hopeful replacements, long-forgotten names such as 'nervous temperament,' 'nervous erethism,' 'mimosis inquieta,' 'cerebro-pathy,' 'cerebral irritation,' 'spinal irritation,' and 'spinal neurosis.' Such names proliferated toward the end of the century, as more and more experiences of dysphoria and deviancy came to be understood as suitable territory for the increasingly expansionist disciplines of neurology, psychiatry, and sexology.

The most significant attempt to reinvent hypochondria came with George Beard's wildly popular diagnosis 'neurasthenia,' a term that started appearing in textbooks through the 1870s and quickly monopolized the medical imagination. By 1902 it was possible for one medical writer to say, 'Neurasthenia used to be called hypochondriasis.' In his 1904 treatise *Die Hypochondrie* the psychiatrist Robert Wollenberg wrote that, in the history of hypochondria, there was a 'pre-neurasthenic' and a 'neurasthenic' period. The importance of this new diagnosis is captured by the historian Esther Fischer-Homberger, who writes that with the appearance of Beard's first book on neurasthenia, the 'Babelic diversity of terminology' was 'reduced to a single term.'

'Neurasthenia' meant nerve weakness. The term was used to describe the psychosomatic symptoms that had become common in US cities in the second half of the nineteenth century. Beard's view was that these nervous phenomena were caused by damage inflicted to the nerves by the strains and stresses of modern life, with the five primary culprits being steam power, the periodical press, the telegraph, the sciences, and the mental activity of women.

The notion that disease had some connection to modernity was not novel. In 1733's *The English Malady*, George Cheyne had argued that hypochondria and hysteria had become endemic to the world capital, making them symptoms of material affluence: 'Since our Wealth has increas'd,' he writes, 'and our Navigation has been extended, we have ransack'd all the Parts of the Globe to bring together its whole Stock of Materials for Riot, Luxury, and to provoke Excess.' Meanwhile in *Diseases of Modern Life* (1876) Benjamin Ward Richardson wrote that the working practices and lifestyles of the nineteenth-century city were producing many harms, including a surge in hypochondria.

Beard took these ideas and used them to elaborate a specifically American new illness, doing so with an evident sense of pride. Where the eighteenth century had been the age of the English malady, the urbanization and economic growth enjoyed by the United States in the years following Reconstruction meant that this was the era of 'American Nervousness,' the title of Beard's bestselling 1881 book.

According to Beard, hypochondria, in the sense of a 'groundless fear of disease,' was in fact extremely rare, and in most cases the diagnosis was used by physicians as 'a cover for our lack of thoroughness in examination.' Beard was himself no stranger to hypochondriac symptoms, as understood at the time: in his late adolescence and early twenties he suffered from tinnitus, fluctuating pain, dyspepsia, nervousness, morbid fears, and 'lack of vitality.' This led him to recognize the importance, particularly among men, of creating a 'legitimate' diagnosis which avoided the pejorative connotations that the old names had started to acquire. By having a physical etiology, grounded in environmental factors, the diagnosis was able to avoid the stigma that had come to be associated with hypochondria.

Neurasthenia conferred many of the advantages of disease – sympathy, time off work, perhaps at a popular convalescent spa – with few of the downsides. Naturally this suited patients. It was also good for doctors. By giving a somatic foundation to nervous disorders, neurasthenia legitimized the expansion of nervous medicine beyond the realm of the asylum. Large cities saw an increasing number of nerve doctors, offering private outpatient services, often to a rarefied professional clientele.

By 1895 William James, who two decades earlier had professed his hypochondria, was calling himself 'a victim of neurasthenia, and of the sense of hollowness and unreality that goes with it.' If modernity was making people sick, then being sick was a way of being modern: before long neurasthenia, like hypochondria a century before, had become a fashionable diagnosis, with brainsick urbanites flocking to nerve doctors and magic mountain–style retreats.

Beard was a canny businessman. He made his neurasthenia diagnosis funnel-like: wide at the top, narrow at the base. In this way he could take an extraordinarily diverse array of clinical and cultural phenomena (fear, fatigue, depression, dizziness, premature balding, disaffection, skin rashes, suicide) and reduce them to a single explanation. However, this superstructural heterogeneity also made the concept structurally unsound: 'To make neurasthenia everything is indeed to make it nothing,' warned Clifford Allbutt in 1910. Sir Andrew Clark – physician to Alice James, William (and Henry's) chronically invalided sister – went further. By purporting to know that 'the whole and sole cause' of such a diverse set of symptoms 'is to be found in this alleged exhaustion,' Beard had committed 'an unpardonable sin' against science. His claims were without foundation: the lesions on which the diagnosis supposedly rested were nowhere to be found. And as biologists continued to identify the microscopic agents of infectious disease, the claim that these lesions were extremely small sounded increasingly evasive.

In the first years of the twentieth century, neurasthenia ceased to provide a coherent explanation for the wide umbrella of symptoms to which it had once provided cover. According to the historian Barbara Sicherman, Beard lost ground on two fronts: on the one hand diagnostic advances made it possible to show that many erstwhile neurasthenics truly suffered from pulmonary tuberculosis, anemia, and endocrine disorders, while on the other Freudian metapsychology began to divide up the territory once monopolized by Beard's concept into the various obsessive, phobic, and depressive states that made up the psychoneuroses. In addition to this, when soldiers began returning from the trenches of the First World War with a range of psychosomatic symptoms, trauma became the major concept in the etiology of nervous illness.

One side effect of all this was to make even more nebulous whatever was named by the word 'hypochondria.' Though it would continue to appear in manuals for some decades to come, neurasthenia ceased to be a common or credible diagnosis. Meanwhile hypochondria, briefly considered obsolete, crossed the threshold of the twentieth century, where it proceeded to continue its strange afterlife as the most thoroughly questionable of illnesses.

The period during which I experienced the most intense fears about my health lasted for five years: from 2010 to 2015. In the course of that period, hypochondria ceased to exist.

The precise moment of this disappearance can be dated to 18 May 2013, when 'hypochondriasis' was removed from the fifth edition of the DSM. As in the case of hysteria three decades earlier, few people mourned the departure of hypochondriasis from the annals of official psychiatry. That said, I for one must confess to a certain fondness for the expurgated term, the incoherence of it, the way its nested reference to rib cartilage serves as a reminder about the limits of knowledge, the risk of misinterpretation underlying every diagnosis.

Since this diagnostic fiat, there have, at least in the view of the American Psychiatric Association, been no hypochondriacs, though it is worth noting that the World Health Organization disagrees. For my part, I did not notice any change when I woke up that Saturday morning, did not register any shift in my symptomatology, in my comorbidity indications.

Today, in place of hypochondriacs stand the sufferers of somatic symptom disorder and, more rarely, illness anxiety disorder. The difference between these two disorders hinges on the respective presence or absence of bodily symptoms. According to 2013's DSM-5, three-quarters of erstwhile hypochondriacs now have somatic symptom disorder while the remaining quarter, those who toil in fear with neither ache nor pain nor trembling heart, suffer from illness anxiety disorder.

This decision was not taken lightly. In 2000 a ten-member 'somatic symptom disorders work group' was established, which would go on to spend more than a decade deliberating as to what to do about hypochondriasis and the broader category of 'somatoform disorders' to which it belonged.

Since 1980, the somatoform disorders had named a group of mental illnesses whose common feature was the presence of 'physical symptoms … for which there are no demonstrable organic findings.' In 1994's DSM-IV there were seven such illnesses, including 'somatization disorder,' the modern successor to the hysteria of Charcot and Freud. The reasons for the move were severalfold. Among them was the view that this category reinforced a Cartesian mind–body dualism, that it was vague, and that names such as 'hypochondriasis' were etymologically incorrect and carried with them a burden of stigma.

Some members of the work group complained that the term 'somatoform,' by combining a Greek prefix with a Latin suffix, was 'difficult to understand' (a view that puts at risk words such as metadata, neuroscience, meritocracy, sociology, and sociopath). Others found that the diagnosis of hypochondriasis had become too restrictive, meaning that, despite its cultural familiarity, in clinical practice it was seldom used. This meant that epidemiological data were unreliable; that, as the authors of one clinical handbook alarmingly put it, 'the true prevalence of hypochondriasis may have been underestimated.'

But there was a bigger problem than each of these: the fact that hypochondriasis and its related disorders had been defined negatively, in relation to the absence of a medical explanation for the patient's somatic symptoms, as in the DSM-IV, which stipulated the failure of a 'thorough' and 'appropriate' medical examination to 'identify a general medical condition.' The problem with basing a diagnosis of hypochondria on the foundation of medically unexplained symptoms was that, as the researchers argued, 'unexplained' could simply mean 'unexamined' – as in the case of Lisa Steen, the doctor who was found to have metastatic cancer having spent years wandering in 'the wilderness of the medically unexplained.'

It's worth remembering that in the twenty-first century the majority of mental illnesses are diagnosed not by a psychiatrist, but by a primary care physician. And so, as Beard was pointing to in the 1880s, the risk is that hypochondria is simply applied to 'difficult' patients – used to conceal a physician's failure to find a physical cause. Indeed in the United States medical error is currently the third most common cause of mortality, accounting for as many as one death in every ten. (The worst thing about writing a book called *Hypochondria* is that it turns out everyone has a story to tell you about an acquaintance, long written off as a hypochondriac, who went on to die from an illness that, caught earlier, they would have survived.)

Meanwhile some diseases may produce symptoms for many years before the underlying cause reveals itself (multiple sclerosis, lupus, certain cancers) while with diseases such as Lyme, chronic fatigue, and fibromyalgia, a definitive pathology might never become manifest. Ultimately, the lack of a physical explanation for the patient's symptoms makes for an unstable foundation for the diagnosis of a mental illness because it is impossible to demonstrate, beyond all doubt, that a person's body is free from disease; and as to what, under such epistemological conditions, constitutes 'reasonable' and 'unreasonable' concern – this amounts to a moral judgment of the sort that, in the twenty-first century, scientific bodies such as the APA do not wish to be seen to be adjudicating on.

What the members of the somatic symptom disorders work group were grappling with was the fact that hypochondria had come to be understood as a form of negativity – or, per Deleuze, 'a negativism beyond all negation.' As they put it in a joint paper, 'medical diagnosis does not usually define a disorder based simply on the absence of something' but 'according to the presence of certain positive features.' The Cartesian attitudes put forward by DSM-IV, with its diagnosis of hypochondriasis (and its roman numerals), were 'more consonant with the 17th century than the 21st.' For this reason, the authors of DSM-5 sought to replace 'the old somatoform perspective' with 'the new category of Somatic Symptom Disorder,' whose diagnosis would not be based on the lack of physical explanations but on the presence of observable psychological phenomena, namely 'disproportionate and excessive thoughts, feelings, and behaviors' relating to symptoms or health concerns.

Like Beard a century before them, the members of the work group were attempting to modernize hypochondria, to bring it into line with contemporary paradigms, so as to put this ancient diagnosis onto a positive, scientific footing.

*

The introduction of the 'somatic symptom and related disorders' turned out to be a cause of considerable controversy, a major episode in a history of hypochondria that, for all its intrigues, has for the most part unfolded outside the purview of the news media. The most vocal critic was Allen Frances, who began sounding the alarm some months before the publication of the new edition.

Something you should know about Allen Frances is that he chaired the group that wrote 1994's DSM-IV, with its diagnosis of hypochondriasis. However, this was not simply the narcissism of minor differences. In fact, the stakes could hardly be higher, since the new guidelines, in his view, risked misdiagnosing vast numbers of people, especially those who were physically sick, with a mental illness. The reason was this: by doing away with the requirement for medically unexplained symptoms, the new diagnosis of somatic symptom disorder shifted the emphasis solely to the patient's attitude regarding somatic symptoms. This meant that, in theory, the new diagnosis could equally apply to those who did in fact have a physical diagnosis to explain their symptoms.

Recall, some patients, about a quarter of those previously labelled 'hypochondriac', experienced anxiety about illness in the complete absence of any physical symptoms; these were the sufferers of the new diagnosis of illness anxiety disorder. But for the majority of former hypochondriacs, the remaining three-quarters, there was in fact the presence of at least one physical symptom; the problem was the 'excessive' thoughts and feelings they attached to it. The rationale for this change was clear enough: psychological and physical symptoms can coexist, and so, with admirable liberalism, the authors of the new edition would refuse to 'question the reality of patients' suffering.' However, because the diagnosis could now apply to anyone, the outcome was that patients with diagnosed physical health conditions were liable to be diagnosed with a comorbid mental illness if they were distressed by their symptoms or by what the future might hold for them.

This was not mere speculation. The over-inclusiveness of the diagnosis was suggested by the new work group's own field studies, which showed that somatic symptom disorder captured 15 percent of patients with cancer or heart disease, 26 percent with irritable bowel syndrome or fibromyalgia, and that it had a high false positive rate of 7 percent among healthy people in the general population.

Under the new framework, there remained what was fundamentally a moral question regarding how much fear or anxiety should be deemed 'excessive.' However, now this question could be applied also, and especially, to the diagnosed sufferers of physical illnesses (thus: the DSM as a sort of conduct manual for appropriate suffering). Where hypochondria had come to be seen as a condition of the worried well, the new disorder seemed likely to disproportionately apply to those who did in fact have a diagnosed physical illness. And aside from these concerns, all of them reasonable, I think it's fair to say that it is difficult to see the wisdom of a diagnostic framework that cannot categorically distinguish between my anxiety regarding the tumour that I do have and my anxiety regarding the tumour that I do not, or might not, have.

As the professor of psychiatry Vladan Starcevic put it, 'When the diagnostic criteria for DSM-IV hypochondriasis were "translated" into those for … DSM-5, some crucial components of hypochondriasis were lost, making the new concepts deficient at best and clinically useless at worst.' It was, Starcevic concludes, 'premature to exclude hypochondriasis from psychiatric nosology.' Such concerns have led many doctors to reject the new terms, and when the WHO published the eleventh edition of the *International Classification of Diseases* (ICD) in 2019, the diagnosis of hypochondriasis remained intact. Perhaps we can simply say that some doctors have come to realize what certain patients have long known: that when it comes to hypochondria, words alone are not enough to banish it. More than a century after Freud, this is the current 'position' of hypochondria: whether one's fears can be called hypochondriac remains a question of whom one asks.

Hypochondria slinks through the medical literature like the Cheshire Cat: that mischievous presence of which nothing remains but the grin. At its simplest, hypochondria names the condition of those who take as a matter of life or death what they know might be nothing at all. How fitting, when you think about it, that no one can agree whether it should be considered an illness.

PRACTICAL CRITICISM

By the autumn of 2010 I have started taking amitriptyline and propranolol, two antidepressant medications that in small doses are used to treat tension headaches, doing so more or less out of politeness, possibly open-mindedness, and probably also in an attempt to appear like a good patient, but without really holding out much hope. And true enough, they have no noticeable effect, aside from causing a mild dyspepsia that, two centuries earlier, could have seen me diagnosed with hypochondria – for which disease I may have been treated, were my class origins more rarefied, by being invited to take the waters at Bath, or Leamington, or Malvern.

If this is a disappointment, then it is one that's shot through with relief: should those strips of tiny blue and yellow pills have worked, I tell myself, possibly only as a result of the placebo effect, then it would have muddled my narrative, putting me in the uncomfortable position of needing to lie to the doctor. Symptoms themselves had never really troubled me. What I wanted was to get beneath experience, to the reality it obscured.

According to modern clinical definitions, hypochondria exists when a patient has fears regarding illness that persist in spite of 'appropriate medical reassurance.' Having examined the patient's body, the doctor finds no evidence to support their concerns. The patient, however, mistrusts the doctor's cool assessment of the facts and thereby becomes a hypochondriac.

Hypochondria, at its core, is an experience of doubt. This might begin in the doctor's office but quickly reaches beyond it, eventually extending to every diagnosis or test that fails to find evidence of serious disease. And yet however much the hypochondriac doubts medical reassurance, they rarely reject the whole enterprise out of hand, since medicine, would it listen, would its official representatives only take notice, tends to constitute the hypochondriac's best and final hope. This is why, however much I doubted what the doctor was saying to me – her insistence that everything I was experiencing could be explained as 'tension' – I continued to find myself in her waiting room, where, always careful to arrive ten minutes early, I would refresh my memory of the past weeks by scrolling through the notes I'd typed on my phone.

*

In its purest form, hypochondria can be expressed as the question: how can I know my body? Or better still: can I know it? I imagine that people have always wondered such things, but this line of inquiry was given new urgency by René Descartes and the methodological doubt and metaphysical dualism he left to the world.

On the evening of 10 November 1619, while he was ensconced in southern Germany during a period of intensive study, the twenty-three-year-old Descartes fell asleep and had a series of three dreams. In the first, he is assailed by phantoms. Attempting to escape, he seeks refuge in a college chapel, where he intends to pray but struggles to gain entry. A missed inter-action with an old friend convinces him to retrace his steps, at which point somebody tries to give him a melon. The wind dies down, and Descartes wakes with a terrible pain in his left side which convinces him that an 'evil demon' is 'trying to deceive him.' Such is the dread produced by this dream that he lies awake for several hours.

In the second dream he hears a thunderclap and sees a shower of bright sparks. Looking about him he observes that he is in his own bedroom. This familiar setting, however, only serves to emphasize a disconcerting fact: Descartes is unable to determine if he is awake or asleep.

In the third, the longest and most elaborate dream, if also the least plausible, the dream that appears to have undergone the heaviest revisions of the conscious mind, Descartes finds a vast tome, an encyclopedia, then another book bearing the words '*Quod vitae sectabor iter?*' ('What road in life shall I follow?'). After that he has a long dialogue with a stranger. Still asleep, Descartes begins interpreting his dream from within, absorbing it into a rather inflated self-mythology: in short, it is up to him to complete the encyclopedia by founding a comprehensive and systematic philosophical science.

Two decades later, while living in the north of Holland, these dreams came back to Descartes as he sat down to write what would go on to become his most famous work.

'Some years ago,' begins the *Meditations*, 'I was struck by the large number of falsehoods that I had accepted as true … and by the highly doubtful nature of the whole edifice that I had sub-sequently based on them.' Descartes then proceeds to search for an indubitable ground for thinking – in his words, 'clear and distinct' knowledge of the truth.

Rather than repudiating doubt, this means accepting it, acceding to it, pushing it to its uppermost limit: it is necessary, he writes, to 'demolish everything completely and start again from the foundations.' Given the way a stick appears to bend when placed in water, how can I trust what my senses tell me? How can I be certain that 'the sky, the air, the earth, colours, shapes, sounds and all external things' are real, and not merely a dream, or else a hallucination induced by some evil power, a 'genius malignus'? How can I know that I exist at all?

Descartes's famous solution lay in the dictum *Cogito, ergo sum*, 'I think, therefore I am.' In the inescapably reflexive nature of doubting lies consciousness itself. Descartes's insight was that, while it's logically possible to doubt the existence of one's body, and even of the entire world, it isn't possible to doubt the reality of this conscious activity of doubting. Having applied the universal solvent of doubt, what is left is the conscious 'I.' On the indubitable ground of the self, Descartes builds his metaphysics, proceeding, through the subsequent meditations, to find evidence for the existence of external reality, God, and free will. Descartes's methodological doubt is therefore an inoculation: with it, he hopes to achieve a degree of certainty immune to any further doubt.

Of course it is not Descartes's legacy to have successfully eradicated doubt from Western intellectual history. In a rapidly secularizing culture, much of what Descartes deemed indubitable – God, the immortality of the soul – would quickly be dispatched with. Meanwhile doubt would increasingly become synonymous with the activity of thinking itself, since, whether due to ideology, slave morality, or repression, first appearances are always, and by their very nature, deceptive.

In spite of Descartes's attempt to banish doubt once and for all, he appears to have unrestrained it. Perhaps it is not surprising, then, that when it came to navigating the social realm, paranoia was his standard protocol: he published under pseudonyms, moved between the cities of the Dutch Republic while concealing his address, and hid his date of birth for fear that some member of the public might take it upon themselves to send him an unsolicited horoscope, whose faulty prognostications, he feared, he would have no option but to believe.

But the greatest effects of doubt were to be experienced when regarding one's own body. For Descartes the mind is a kind of theatre in which sensations are paraded before an inner eye. What this inner eye sees are not things, therefore, but representations. And so, with Descartes a previously unthinkable question now becomes urgent: how does the mind know the world? Or: (how) do we know that our thoughts and feelings reflect anything real? More troubling still, though the mind is 'dependent upon the condition and relation of the organs of the body,' mind and body now occupy completely separate spheres of reality; and though the mind can know itself – 'Nothing is easier for the mind to know but itself' – the body in which it is housed becomes a dubious entity whose every sensation is questionable.

Descartes himself displayed a deep concern about the state of his body. Of 'all the blessings of this life,' he writes in *Discourse on the Method*, 'the preservation of health … is without doubt … the first and fundamental one.' A scientific optimist, Descartes believed that we will 'free ourselves from an infinity of maladies of body as well as of mind' once we have 'sufficiently ample knowledge of their causes.' Descartes did not believe that animals had any moral value but was a committed vegetarian who sustained himself on the plants from his own garden in the belief that he might live to a hundred. However, illness was never far from mind – that of his mother, who died a year after he was born, and his own: 'From her I inherited a dry cough and a pale colour which stayed with me until I was more than twenty, so that all the doctors who saw me up to that time condemned me to die young.'

If Descartes was by turns anxious and optimistic about the state of his health, then this attitude was, in a sense, the logical outcome of his philosophy. The mind is housed inside a body from which it is always estranged. That body is a machine, and therefore optimizable. But it is also a foreign entity that is fundamentally unknowable. The philosopher Gilbert Ryle famously summed up Descartes's mind-body dualism with the phrase 'the ghost in the machine.' But in the anxious metaphysics that Descartes left us, and under whose shadow we still live, it is the ghost that is haunted by the machine.

'Strictly speaking, there is no science of health,' writes the philosopher Georges Canguilhem. 'Health is organic innocence. It must be lost, like all innocence, so that knowledge may be possible.' If health is a form of innocence, a sort of unselfconscious flourishing, then what does this mean for an era of ever-extending knowledge about disease? What happens to health in societies that are concerned, precisely, with health?

In premodern times, disease adhered closely to the subjective experience of illness. This is because there were only very limited tools for distinguishing the latent and the manifest: to be sick was to feel unwell. Across the Enlightenment the two steadily begin parting ways, but the seismic shift occurred in the second half of the nineteenth century, with the development of X-rays and microbiology, technologies that broke the old alliance between eye and world by making it possible to see the invisible vectors and lesions of disease. Like Descartes, the pioneers of these technological developments laid bare the chasm between experience and reality: increasingly disease was something that could exist in the body without erupting into consciousness.

In industrialized countries over the last century and half, developments in medicine, sanitation, and hygiene mean that the landscape of death has been transformed beyond recognition. For a hundred years between 1750 and 1850 UK life expectancy hovered at around forty. Across the same span, between 1850 and 1950, it rose from forty to sixty-eight, reaching eighty-one by 2020. In 1908 a third of deaths were in under-fives; today that figure is less than one in a hundred. In 1908 fewer than one person in ten would live to seventy-five; today fewer than one in three will die before reaching that age.

Changes with regards to who is dying have been accompanied and abetted by changes to how people are dying. In 1908 infectious disease accounted for 20 percent of deaths; today (with a brief anomaly in 2020–21) it accounts for 7 percent. Across the same period, deaths caused by chronic, progressive diseases have steadily increased. In 1908 cancer was responsible for around one death in twenty, while heart disease did not cause statistically significant mortality; by 1948 these two diseases had become the main cause of death in England and Wales. In 1901 Alzheimer's disease was first observed and named; in the ten years between 2012 and 2021, Alzheimer's and other dementias were the leading cause of death in the UK. Death no longer bursts in rudely on the scene of life; it advances slowly, tactfully, governed by a set of recognizable customs.

One effect of all this has been to assign a new role to the notion of 'awareness.' In 1907 the surgeon and early cancer activist Charles Childe published *The Control of a Scourge, Or How Cancer Is Curable*, addressed to a general readership. In it he warns, 'You measure your disease by the amount of suffering it causes you, a natural but ghastly error.' This means that cancer's innocent victims are often 'quite naturally lulled by the entire absence of symptoms into a sense of security … All the time this terrible crab is fixing its murderous seed, its unlucky victim feels perfectly well, and imagines himself to be so.' Axiomatic to Childe's book was the idea that 'Cancer itself is not incurable. It becomes incurable from the simple fact that its unfortunate victims harbour and nurse their cancers till it is too late.' For this reason Childe devoted himself to publicizing the 'earliest manifestations of the disease' in order to banish the 'ignorance of which we see every day is fraught with such terrible consequences.'

In the decades that followed, innocence would become one of the greatest threats to a person's physical well-being. Starting in the 1930s, cancers that respond better to treatment before they have become very advanced – at a period during which any manifestations are discreet and quotidian – become a frequent topic of public information campaigns, aided by the rise of mass media. In the United States, the American Society for the Control of Cancer (the forerunner of the American Cancer Society) delivered the message that 'Delay Kills!' Between 1936 and 1948 a 'Women's Field Army,' kitted out in khaki, informed the public about the value of smear tests, clinical and self-performed breast exams, and practicing vigilance toward early warning signs. In this 'fight,' the Society deployed the weapons of a growing publicity industry: a WWII–era poster claimed that more people died each fortnight from a delayed cancer diagnosis than had died at Pearl Harbor.

In the decades since then, awareness campaigns have become commonplace. A few years ago I remember seeing posters around London warning 'You can't always see the signs' and encouraging people to check their stools for early signs of bowel cancer. In 2022, a charity displayed a billboard image of a pair of pendulous testes with the caption, 'Have you checked yours this month?' Or, for dementia: 'Forgetting where they put the car is one thing. Not being able to remember whether it's blue, red, silver or white is another entirely.' These sorts of campaigns publicise the gap between subjective experience and organic reality: between how well you might feel and how sick you might be.

In this gap there is also a lot of money to be made. Since the late 1990s, websites such as WebMD and Healthline have grown into multimillion-dollar businesses by disseminating lists of early warning signs. 'Did you know your nails can reveal clues to your overall health?' begins a typical article on WebMD. These articles tend to emphasise the arbitrariness of the relationship between signifier and signified: 'A touch of white here, a rosy tinge there, or some rippling or bumps may be a sign of disease in the body. Problems in the liver, lungs, and heart can show up in your nails. Keep reading to learn what secrets your nails might reveal.' All this makes for pretty compelling copy, at least for the right sort of reader, which is obviously important for a business model that works by monetizing attention. The success of these companies indicates a shift in reading habits: where in the twentieth century health organizations used the tools of the advertising industry to publicise health risks, today private companies publicize health risks to sell consumer products.

In *The Semiotic Challenge* Roland Barthes reminds us that the word *semiology* originally applied to the reading not of literature but of the first and most perplexing text: the human body. These campaigns and articles are an exercise in practical criticism. They train people to be suspicious readers of their bodies. Today, merely feeling well is not enough – and if anything, is slightly irresponsible. To be truly healthy, one must be more critical with regard to one's experience of subjective well-being. A sunken nail bed? A headache? A sore? How long has this mild cough been going on? Did I always become so bloated after dinner? Don't my gums bleed each time I brush my teeth?

Organic innocence, replaced by knowledge. Canguilhem's postlapsarian metaphor to describe health might serve to remind us of the religious roots of the concept of this word, which is etymologically related to 'whole' and 'holy.' These roots are visible in the WHO's phantasmatic definition of health as 'state of complete physical, mental and social well-being and not merely the absence of disease or infirmity.' Under contemporary conditions the ideal of perfect health becomes something of a self-contradicting enterprise, since the only way it can be ensured is through a practice of conscious scrutiny that is incompatible with any holistic ideal. In the words of Wendell Berry:

> From our constant and increasing concerns about health, you can tell how seriously diseased we are. Health, as we may remember from at least some of the days of our youth, is at once wholeness and a kind of unconsciousness. Disease (dis-ease), on the contrary, makes us conscious not only of the state of our health but of the division of our bodies and our world into parts.

Perhaps this is really what Freud meant when he said that hypochondria exposes the limits of our knowledge. Not an absence of knowledge, a gap that could be filled with new information, but a more categorical deficiency: the failure of knowledge to ever bring about the states of health, happiness, or even certainty which we prefer.

Simone Weil considered 'Why am I being hurt?' to be the most fundamental human question, 'the childish cry which Christ himself could not restrain.' Suffering, one can't help but wonder why. Happy, most people tend to just go with it, to see where it takes them, which means that happiness, like health, is difficult to catch in flight. However, this entails a degree of abandonment that hypochondriacs can't endure. Hence the dialectical traps in which they're liable to ensnare themselves: the hypochondriac wants to feel healthy, vibrant, alive, yet in their desire to be certain of these things, they constantly find themselves feeling the opposite.

'Ours is an age which consciously pursues health, and yet only believes in the reality of sickness,' writes Susan Sontag. Health has become elusive in a society in which people are encouraged to scrutinize all aspects of their mental and bodily well-being: today being well means forever wondering just how 'well' one really is.

On Saturday 6 August 1763 a twenty-two-year-old James Boswell arrived at Harwich, where he boarded the Prince of Wales. Disembarking near Rotterdam the following day, he made his way toward Utrecht where at the behest of his father he was to spend the year studying law. A funereal air descended as the young hedonist was carried by horse-drawn barge – at an agonizingly slow pace, as if against the will of nature – into the quiet university city that was for the foreseeable future to be his new home.

A few days earlier, everything had been different. His revered friend Samuel Johnson had accompanied Boswell to Harwich, and while he understood the gravity of the next year, so long as it was still over the horizon, he was not blind to its possibilities: 'Resolve now study in earnest,' he wrote in a note to himself, dated 1 August. 'Consider you're not to be so much a student as a traveller. Be a liberal student. Learn to be reserved. Keep your melancholy to yourself, and you'll easily conceal your joy.' Those thoughts were a long way off now, however, as were the memories of the happy hours he spent conversing with Johnson as the pair made their way from London to Essex.

On arrival to the city, he was shown to his new lodgings. From his upstairs room, he was appalled by the loud tolling of the church bell. The thought that he would hear this same 'dreary psalm tune' twenty-four times a day, for the next ten months, must have felt like a cruel metaphor for the monotony that lay in store.

'A deep melancholy seized me,' he wrote to his friend John Johnston some weeks later. 'I groaned with the idea of living all winter in so shocking a place ... I was worse and worse the next day. All the horrid ideas that you can imagine, recurred upon me.' Despondency soon gave way to more heated feelings:

'I ran frantic up and down the streets, crying out, bursting into tears, and groaning from my innermost heart.'

The bright side of all this was that it made him more like Johnson, who a few weeks earlier had told him that he, too, often found himself 'greatly distressed.' Perhaps recalling that conversation, Boswell turned to one of Johnson's *Rambler* essays, which he took to be 'describing the wretchedness of a mind unemployed.' His friend Temple supported that diagnosis, telling Boswell 'your sole disease is idleness.' Soon Boswell had recomposed himself: 'I began to think that I had no title to shelter myself from blame under the excuse of madness which was perhaps but a suggestion of idle imagination.' Resolving, there and then, to 'harden himself against being unhinged by little evils,' he decided he would fix himself down to 'a regular plan, and to persist with firmness and spirit, and combat the foul fiend.'

In Boswell's journals and correspondence, this foul fiend went by several names: melancholy, spleen, and hypochondria. Over time, the latter became his preferred term, and when, years later, he authored a series of periodical essays in the Johnsonian style, it was under the pseudonym 'the Hypochondriack.'

In Holland Boswell's plan for banishing his hypochondria consisted of the attempt to keep himself occupied at all times, to plan, and thus account for, every waking moment. He wrote daily memoranda, addressing himself in the second person as he set out in painstaking detail the tasks to be performed and the moral qualities embodied in the hours that lay ahead:

> Latin till breakfast, something till eleven, then dress and at twelve French, then walk and dine. Afternoon, journal, &c ... Mem. worthy father. Guard against liking

billiards. They are blackguard … Be easy and natural, though a little proud. Write out full mem. that this is your winter to get rid of spleen and become a man.

As Brian Dillon points out, Boswell's mania for planning is taken so far that 'his plans even contain, as here, reminders to copy out further plans.' It is as if he feared that a single moment unaccounted for, a single gap in his daily routine, would be enough space to allow the foul fiend to steal its way back into his life.

As the weeks pass, there is an increasingly harried tone in the memoranda, which, even at their most exuberant, give the impression of a mind on the verge of collapse. Addressing himself, Boswell has little time for niceties; his standard grammatical mood is the imperative: 'Read your Plan every morning regularly at breakfast … Get commonplace-book … Be steady' (16 October). 'Never aim at being too brilliant. Be rather an amiable, pretty man. Have no affection. Cure vanity … Take exercise. Be independent' (19–20 December). 'Starve and keep off spleen' (21 December).

Before long, he is not simply looking ahead at the day to come, but also looking back his previous day's performance, rereading it in the harsh morning light: 'Yesterday you was very splenetic … Dined ordinary. Then idle. Billiards by self' (1 January). 'Yesterday you was lethargic and still hippish and gaunt … You are not really well at present' (22 February).

Plans to socialize rarely appear in his morning memoranda, and yet however pure his intentions, when he comes to review the previous day, Boswell constantly finds that he has been out drinking, being his least preferred version of himself – simpering, loose, and braggart. 'Yesterday you … talked too bold on

Inquisition, &c., though you want knowledge' (12 May), 'You talked too much in vivacious style to Rose, and a little too much to Guiffardiere' (19 October), 'Yesterday you was still too jocular and talked of yourself, particularly of your whoring, which was shameful' (23 October), 'Yesterday you deviated sadly ... In the evening you resolved to bring up journal; and instead of that you sat seven hours at cards' (7 January).

This is not to suggest that Boswell never has a kind word himself – 'You did charmingly yesterday. You attended well to everything' (28 October) – and yet even when he does, there is often a hint of reproach, perhaps as a warning against the temptations of vanity, pride, and complacency ('You did very well yesterday, only you transgressed a little in talking of yourself' [22 October]), and reading these memoranda there is the uncomfortable looming sense that Boswell is just one little slip, just a single mishap or misadventure away from letting the whole thing fall apart. 'Yesterday you did not at all keep to rules as you ought to,' begins a typical entry. Invariably his solution is stricter rules, fewer distractions, harder study – as if he were forever but a single good day's reading from acquiring the discipline and insight that would save him.

Boswell was no stranger to health concerns, especially regarding the venereal disease that was to be his clandestine companion – 'all night, I lay in direful apprehension that my testicle, which formerly was ill, was again swelled' (4 February 1763) – but for him hypochondria primarily named something else. His fear of moral and physical collapse, but also the obsession with discipline and order with which he tried to combat it, this strange convergence of self-cure and symptom. Read cumulatively, this carousel of relapses and resolutions forms a tragicomic record of a self that is constantly getting away from itself.

'A man should not live more than he can record,' Boswell once wrote, though given his taste for living, in practice this meant that each day he had to spend several hours at his desk, bringing his journal up to date, pen in hand as he tried desperately to keep pace with himself. It was a habit he had begun in London a year earlier, and which he would continue for the rest of his life.

But everything we know of this unhappy period in Holland is what can be pieced together from bits of ephemera: Boswell's daily memoranda, as well as his French and Dutch writing exercises, and his always garrulous correspondence. The journal itself was lost during his own lifetime. When he left Utrecht in June 1764, he packed up his papers and delivered them to his friend the Reverend Robert Brown, to be forwarded to him in Scotland after his return from his European tour. Brown seems to have entrusted them to a young army officer, who carried them back in his cloak bag. But when the papers were finally delivered, the journal was missing. No good explanation was ever found; it had simply gone the way of lost things. This would upset anyone. But for Boswell, to whom the unrecorded life was not worth living, was in fact barely life at all, the loss must have been alarming, a chilling foretaste of death.

Not long before he died, Kafka wrote a brief text which Max Brod later named 'The Top.' The narrative concerns a philosopher who is convinced that busying oneself with 'great problems' is uneconomical; 'the understanding of any detail,' he believes, 'that of a spinning top, for instance,' is 'sufficient for the understanding of all things.' And so 'whenever he saw a boy with a top, he would lie in wait,' and try to 'catch the top while it was still spinning.' Here are the final lines:

> And whenever preparations were being made for the spinning of the top, he hoped that this time it would succeed: as soon as the top began to spin and he was running breathlessly after it, the hope would turn to certainty, but when he held the silly piece of wood in his hand, he felt nauseated. The screaming of the children, which hitherto he had not heard and which now suddenly pierced his ears, chased him away, and he tottered like a top under a clumsy whip.

Across these lines there is a change in verb aspects, from past habitual ('whenever...,' 'the hope would... ') to the simple past ('he felt nauseated...,' 'he tottered like a top... '). So that at its climax, the story takes us from an infernal 'whenever' to the abrupt awakening of 'now.' To be caught in the grips of a repetition compulsion, Kafka's story is suggesting, is to perennially forget (and painfully recall) the machinic patterning of one's behaviour: each time one hopes it will be 'the' time.

Kafka's philosopher is in awe of the animating motion of the spinning top, wishing to grasp it. In this sense he suffers from what Franz Rosenzweig calls *apoplexia philosophica*. In the *Theaetetus*, Plato puts forward the view that philosophy begins with the experience of wonder. However, rejoins Rosenzweig in *Understanding the Sick and the Healthy*, the philosopher is not merely enthralled by but 'addicted to the ways of wonder.' The non-philosopher is content to 'submit' to wonder. Lovers, for instance, 'are no longer a wonder to each other; they are in the heart of wonder.' The children in Kafka's story, this is where they are as well. Meanwhile the person suffering from *apoplexia philosophica*, writes Rosenzweig, wishes to possess wonder, to seize it from the outside.

'The philosopher,' according to the critic Eric Santner (he is writing specifically of Kafka's story), 'appears to be in thrall to the fantasy that the universal principle he seeks can be attained from a position outside the everyday activities that make up a human life.' I think of Kafka's story recently as an old schoolfriend shows me the smartphone app with which he 'tracks' his steps, sleep, and calories. Not a philosopher, he nevertheless appears to have fallen under the authority of the famous Socratic dictum about the unexamined life. Scrolling back through months of accumulated data, he guiltily accounts for any anomalies (holiday, sick leave) in what, if the numbers are telling a reliable story, appears to be an impeccably regulated existence. The app, he finally explains (he is no more specific than this), is providing him with 'insights.'

There are hundreds of these apps and devices on the market, and because my conversation with the old friend piqued my curiosity, prompting online investigations, I have spent several months being aggressively marketed them. So far I have resisted buying one, yet I have come to fully understand their appeal. Take Daily Life Tracker, with its slogan 'Change your habits, change your life.' Who could fail to be stirred by that gamefully leveraged command, requiring only a little input of effort now while promising to yield nothing less than total transformation. This is precisely what Boswell hoped to achieve in Holland, with the tools at his disposal.

These digital technologies grew out of the Quantified Self movement of the early 2010s, whose proponents promised to deliver 'self-knowledge through numbers.' The 'dominant forms of self-exploration assume that the road to knowledge lies through words,' explains founder Gary Wolf. He and his followers, meanwhile, 'are exploring an alternate route. Instead of interrogating their inner worlds through talking and writing, they are using numbers.' If Wolf's millenarian bombast feels a little anachronistic, it is only because tracking apps and devices have become so thoroughly mainstream. Most smartphones track their owners' steps and calories without any prompting. In 2022 the global 'wearable technology' market was valued at $61.3 billion, and from 2023 to 2030 it is forecast to expand at a compound annual growth rate of nearly 15 percent.

Behind these devices lurks the Cartesian notion of the body as a machine, the promise to bring the wayward body back under the authority of the mind. Yet these devices aren't simply more accurate tools for 'quantifying' one's self; they open up new, previously unexamined areas of their users' lives, making them available to analysis and optimisation. One service, which has been given the amiable and teacherly name 'Zoe,' promises to 'map' its user's 'unique' gut biome. This involves wearing a continuous glucose monitor, hitherto reserved for diabetics, so that you can track your glucose level at all points throughout the day. A 'community' of users who, one assumes, had previously little considered their glucose level are now alerted each time it drops or spikes outside an optimal range.

As somebody who often has trouble sleeping, who has sometimes dreamed of writing a serious, scholarly study of insomnia, it is sleep trackers that interest me the most. The current Fitbit allows users to set a 'sleep schedule' (tempting to one who is constantly missing that appointment) while providing 'sleep insights' and a daily 'sleep score.'

Sleep has had a fairly minor place in the history of ideas. Freud describes it as a form of benign narcissism, the nightly withdrawal of worldly investments. Meanwhile, the philosopher Jean-Luc Nancy describes this retreat into one's own self as the discovery of an otherness within:

> By falling asleep, I fall inside myself … I now belong only to myself, having fallen into myself and mingled with that night where everything becomes indistinct to me but more than anything myself … [M]ore than anything, I myself become indistinct … So it is another who sleeps in my place.

David Hume related sleep to fever and madness. Indeed what could be a greater embarrassment to our fantasies of self-possession? Or to the idea of humans as productive consumers? Darian Leader has written perceptively about the paradoxical place of sleep in contemporary culture. 'On the one hand,' he argues, 'we inhabit an unsleeping world of commerce and information, and on the other, we are increasingly told to get the right number of hours of good uninterrupted sleep.' The two are incompatible, he writes, and it's 'in the space opened up by these contradictory imperatives that a lot of money can be made.' Whether in the form of apps, gadgets, books, or pills, the promise is always the same: to reprogram your sleep to optimize it for a world of capitalist competition. It is therefore perhaps not surprising that many large companies now offer their employees free sleep trackers as a form of 'incentivization,' while some go a step further by financially compensating employees whose trackers prove them to be practicing responsible sleep 'hygiene.'

In *24/7: Late Capitalism and the Ends of Sleep*, Jonathan Crary memorably describes capitalism's anxious assaults on sleep. This assault will be a fait accompli once everyone is using one of the sleep trackers between which I am currently being asked to choose. In the end, however, this won't really be because they are keeping to their schedule, hitting high scores and impressing their bosses. It will be because, by continuing to produce data all through the night, users – themselves, of course, 'the product' – will untiringly feed a machine whose appetite remains unsated twenty-four hours a day, seven days a week. And if, as is widely reported, these apps should in fact disrupt one's sleep, turning it into a source of anxiety, then (as those without an ad blocker will no doubt learn soon enough) there are plenty of technological fixes for that malaise.

In *Sex, Or the Unbearable*, Lee Edelman and Lauren Berlant write that the core insight of psychoanalysis is the 'subject's constitutive division that keeps us, as subjects, from fully knowing or being in control of ourselves' – the insight against which James Boswell so valiantly, and so vainly, fought. Against this view, tracking devices promise to fill in the gaps in our self-knowledge; they promise to eliminate doubt as they bring into consciousness every aspect of one's bodily existence. It's easy to see the appeal of the self-possession promised by these devices. They offer a sort of painless vivisection. But as with the children's game in Kafka's story, the things that make up a life are only meaningful from within, incapable of being dissected and grasped by an externalizing logic. In *The Undying*, Anne Boyer calls this 'enchantment' – the 'ordinary magic of all that exists existing for its own sake.'

It is easy to see how in the attempt to lead this version of the examined life one could end up succumbing to *apoplexia philosophica*: as new tracking devices open up more and more areas of one's life to examination, they reveal new gaps in our knowledge of our bodies, which in turn creates the appetite for new devices, feeding an endless cycle.

'Is it possible to conceive a human being with more perfect health than myself?' Kant is said to have exclaimed one evening, swaddled in a blanket, 'self-involved like the silk-worm in its cocoon.' But this equilibrium was hard-won. Looking back over his life in one of his final works, Kant claimed to have cured his own 'natural disposition to hypochondria' through sheer force of will, having tamed his fears about a 'flat and narrow chest, which leaves little room for the movement of the heart and lungs.'

At a time when hypochondria was generally regarded to be a disease of the nerves, Kant comes close to a modern psychological view as he goes on to write that 'though some sort of unhealthy condition ... may be the source of it, this state is not felt immediately, as it affects the senses, but is misrepresented as impending illness by inventive imagination.' Similarly, according to the DSM, the hypochondriac's concern is 'not the somatic symptoms per se,' but 'the way they interpret them.' It's as if the hypochondriac were unable to experience the body directly, only doing so through the mirrored hallway of the mind, with its endless possibilities for distortion and misrepresentation. What obsesses the hypochondriac isn't so much the body itself, but the meanings that it might contain, as if the mind is unable to allow the body to simply 'be' without trying to decipher it.

Where modern mainstream psychiatry tends to view this under the rubric of anxiety, psychoanalysis has tended to view hypochondria as being on a spectrum with paranoia. It's easy to see the connection – in both conditions everyday life is subjected to doubt, interpretation, and an overriding compulsion to know – though it's worth noting that where paranoia can embroil its subject in political or cosmological intrigue, placing them at the centre of vast plots, hypochondriacs tend to be of a more parochial cast, with a zone of interest that generally stops at the outer limits of their bodies.

In her celebrated essay 'Paranoid Reading and Reparative Reading,' the critic Eve Kosofsky Sedgwick analyses paranoia as a style of reading. The paranoiac seeks to close the gap between the apparent meaning of experience and its real meaning, to pass from surface into depth. Sedgwick reveals the contradiction at the heart of paranoia, the way it claims to doubt everything it sees while placing a huge degree of trust in the efficacy of doubt itself, its ability to see through illusion. This, argues Sedgwick, is why paranoid fantasists can be at once doggedly suspicious and oddly credulous, able, for all their scrupulosity, to entertain fantasies of having monopolized Truth.

If we can think of hypochondria as a style of reading, then compared to paranoia, its hold on matters is fairly tenuous. Hypochondria is a form of doubt that has doubts about itself. Its sufferers are not zealots. Perhaps one is simply making it all up, worrying over nothing: these insights are generally available to the hypochondriac, and in addition to the guilty conscience this instills, the feeling of bad faith, it means that one cannot sink into hypochondria like a delusion or suffer it like a fever because to suffer from hypochondria is to wonder if one truly is suffering.

The hypochondriac might like to imagine themselves to be like Descartes – to be exercising a rational faculty of doubt that is confident in its ability to arrive at certainty. But in comparison to Enlightenment philosophers and paranoiacs, hypochondriacs tend to be a little less sure of themselves, a little warier. In this sense, the position of the hypochondriac resembles that of the narrator of Flaubert's 'Memoirs of a Madman,' who after looking back over his life, examining it from every angle, finds that looked at this closely, it no longer makes any sense. In the end he realizes that he can't distinguish reason from madness. Reason is a form of questioning that can only operate if it does so without exception, and so at some point it has to discover that it would be unreasonable to go on taking itself for granted: 'Madness is the doubt of reason. Perhaps it is reason. Who can prove it one way or the other?'

Who can prove it either way? The hypochondriac question par excellence, addressed to the empty space where proofs falter.

*

'To have great pain,' writes Elaine Scarry, is 'to is to have certainty; to hear that another person has pain is to have doubt.' In the case of my headache, the pain was not that great. There were times when I'd forget all about it, the way you don't feel your soles pressing into the ground with every footstep, or how you don't hear your own voice each time you speak: those little ways in which even the most vigilant among us are always slipping away from ourselves. Of course even these things can feel weird when put under conscious scrutiny. Was that it, had I just paid it too much attention? I was sure I could feel something – but was it pain? Perhaps this sensation was really just a presence, a sort of fullness.

Although I didn't say anything about this to anyone, hardly even admitting it to myself, as the months passed I came to doubt whether the headache was really there after all – if what I was experiencing wasn't really just the typically overlooked baseline weird feeling of having a head.

As time passed I started viewing my life through microscopical eyes. I was looking for signs. This was restless work from which even sleep no longer provided respite. Each time I approached the threshold of consciousness I would jolt awake with a surge of electricity in my skull. It was clear this sensation signalled the start of an oncoming seizure; I lay in wait, it didn't come.

Often I would smell smoke. However, I knew that phantom smells were a common (or at least a well-known) symptom of a brain tumour, and so it would therefore be more accurate to say that often I asked myself whether I could smell smoke, while wondering if these weren't really phantom phantom smells, the figments of a hypochondriac imagination. Who could prove it either way? Which is to say that what troubled me wasn't only the question of whether, objectively speaking, there was a fire, but whether subjectively I could smell one. If not, what would it mean to 'believe' I could? Would that even make sense? So then I could smell smoke, purely because the question had arisen? But nothing could be less certain.

On one such occasion I was at work. Looking up from my computer, I asked my colleagues if they could smell anything. At the time I was living in Brighton, finishing up my degree while working as a corporate copywriter. Most of my friends had moved on by now, left the city for London, and it's true that things were worse that year. In this workplace, a fire would have been an appealing thing. It would have distinguished the Tuesday that it was from the Monday it had just been. My question generated a little office murmur, therefore, some inquisitive sniffing of the air, but it was to the shared disappointment of all that no one else could smell anything out of the ordinary.

At such moments I would usually disregard my senses. I'd got used to such tricks, and the sensation in question was rarely strong enough to merit conviction. But I decided on this occasion that I would not be so easily swayed. I walked around the office, peering out of each window. A few people looked on with interest but this did not unsettle me. Intensifying my search, I took the elevator up to the top of the building and started scanning the city below. And sure enough, in the distance, there it was: a column of smoke made picturesque by the late afternoon sun. It was maybe three miles away, where the outer fringes of Kemptown faded into villages whose names I never learned. At such a distance it wasn't possible to see what it was – a house fire that had been brought under control, or just someone burning rubbish in their back garden. The moment struck me as significant, maybe symbolic. But whether it was cause for relief or concern, I wasn't able to say.

*M*ac and His Problem by the Spanish writer Enrique Vila-Matas is an essayistic novel – really, a novelistic essay – about repetition. When he is four years old, a teacher tells the narrator Mac that his friend Soteras will be repeating his preschool year. From that day on, as the other boys age, it is as though Soteras remains frozen in time, and Mac, now in his sixties, is still haunted by the image of 'little Soteras's sad face,' the 'gray cape he wore in winter,' and, above all, by 'his status as a repeater.'

'For many years,' writes Mac, 'Soteras having to repeat the preschool year remained a great enigma to me.' Until, as an adult, he happens to meet him on a bus. Wasting no time, Mac asks him straight out why he had repeated the one 'year that no one ever repeats, namely, the preschool year.' Unfazed, Soteras is only too happy to answer this question, and in fact seems to have been expecting it. '"You won't believe it," he said, "but I asked my parents to let me stay down a year because I was afraid of moving up to the next one."' For Mac this explanation is plausible, banal even, since fear is often what keeps us locked in cycles of repetition. But then Soteras continues:

> Soteras asked if I'd ever heard of someone going to see a movie twice, and entirely failing to understand it the second time around. I stood rooted to the spot, dumbstruck, in the middle of that crowded bus.
>
> 'Well,' he said, 'that's what happened to me after spending two years in preschool: the first time I understood everything, the second time nothing at all.'

*

At graduate school I heard a story about Samuel Beckett, who in response to an audience member asking what one of his stories meant, simply reread it in its entirety. (The story could be apocryphal, or I might be misremembering, I've never been able to verify it.) The gesture was arrogant, declared a classmate who liked to declare things. But the gesture could be read in another way, I felt, not as a rebuke but a heuristic. This way the anecdote becomes a sort of koan, a piece of practical meditation, like the Buddha's flower sermon. As if to suggest, in the gentle, mocking way of a Zen master: if you want to know what a text means, the best thing you can do is to reread it.

I often find myself rereading certain books, though I don't really know why, what I'm looking for. The way I was taught to read was a version of the close reading developed by the New Critics in the 1940s, now broadly unfashionable, though still a mainstay of contemporary humanities departments. The New Critics were a group of male cultural conservatives, mostly at southern US universities, who emphasized the total autonomy of the text – its independence from authorial intent (the 'intentional fallacy'), reader response (the 'affective fallacy'), as well as cultural and political contexts. Through a close and sustained practice of attention to nothing more than the words on the page, the critic sought to clarify the inner workings of the text as an aesthetic totality.

Drawing on *Practical Criticism* by I. A. Richards, the New Critics were seeking to establish a science of reading. Above all, the critic had to keep himself out of the text. The truths produced by close reading were to be social truths, and in theory, universalizable; everyone who paid a text close enough attention ought to come away with the same insights.

Of course the production of universal truths is rarely an unproblematic endeavour, and it seems especially ill-fated as applied to literature. Yet taken as an injunction to a particular exercise of attention, not as an absolute value, the one way to read, I do think the methodology of close reading remains useful. Still, it's no surprise that the New Critics applied plenty of prejudices of their own, among which was their well-known preference for harmony and order, for well-wrought urns. It therefore became an article of faith that what the practice of close reading would reveal was the formal unity of the literary text, the integration of each of its elements, thus elevating it to a higher coherence.

It was while I was learning to read that I was also busy becoming a hypochondriac, treating my body like a work of literature, reading it and rereading it. The headache that might not have been a headache, but also every other little sensation: it seemed like any aspect of experience could become suggestive when I turned my mind toward it. It didn't matter that none of these symptoms were particularly bad – not painful, debilitating, or even significant in themselves – since from browsing online symptomologies, I had come to understand the arbitrariness of the bodily sign: the discoloured nail bed that signifies death.

In 'Against Interpretation,' Susan Sontag decried what she called a 'modern style of interpretation' which believes 'manifest content must be probed and pushed aside to find the true meaning – the latent content beneath.' That's exactly what I wanted, to get beneath experience, to reveal what was hidden. This meant viewing my body with the sort of attention the New Critics reserved for Keats or Shakespeare. I must have been doing something badly wrong, however, because the closer

I looked, the more incoherent things seemed, the less confidently I found myself able to say what it all meant.

The critic D. A. Miller describes something similar happening with the texts to which he returns most frequently (the novels of Jane Austen and the films of Alfred Hitchcock). He reads them, again and again, and as he does so his eye latches onto details that are so slight that he can't be quite sure they're there at all. As Miller writes about Hitchcock, the closer he has looked, the more he has come to suspect that each of his films contains a 'radical duplicity,' as though it had been 'fashioned to conceal something that – if ever seen – would not enhance its coherence, but explode it.'

With a wink, Miller calls this practice too-close reading. Miller's too-close reader has taken some of the New Critical imperatives to heart yet finds they don't produce the proclaimed results. Far from deciphering the text, the too-close reader finds themselves transfixed by meanings that might be meaningless, details that flicker and effervesce. 'None of this, I knew, had any narrative reality,' Miller tells us about his microscopic analysis of one of Hitchcock's films, describing how, as 'the sighter of the unimportant, and indeed the anti-important,' he finds himself beset 'by disagreeable feelings of solitude and isolation.' Eventually, he writes, the question arises: 'Am I the only one?'

Likewise, the hypochondriac remains transfixed by the vanishing point where reality meets imagination, where the subtleties of sensation disappear into naught. In Charlotte Brontë's *Villette*, Lucy Snowe visits the theatre one evening when the king is also in attendance. As she turns away from the diverting public entertainment on stage, she finds herself captivated by the private drama that is unfolding upon his face. Reading the 'hieroglyphics graven ... on his brow,' Lucy recognizes that, below the surface of his cheerful expression, the king is a fellow 'sufferer ... of that strangest spectre, Hypochondria.' Lucy's own hypochondria provides the insight, lost upon everyone else, to whom 'its peculiarity seemed to be wholly invisible.' However, a question remains unsettled regarding what Lucy herself might be bringing to the text. Is the darkness she detects in the king's face really there? Or is it merely her own shadow that is falling across the page?

Doesn't all reading involve these sorts of spectres, this following after what might not be there at all? This is what Maurice Blanchot is suggesting when he writes that reading is a search, but that it is one where one can never quite say what one is looking for, or indeed whether it 'corresponds to anything real, anything possible or anything important.'

Blanchot, the interminable rereader, the critic whose large body of work circles around the same handful of texts (by Mallarmé, Rilke, and above all by Kafka), which he returns to time and again, for five decades, as he seeks the 'essence of literature,' which, he writes, 'is disappearance.' This ghostly condition seemed to follow Blanchot into his personal life. Friends and acquaintances describe him as 'translucent,' a 'diaphanous apparition.' The laconic biographical note accompanying his books said his 'life is entirely devoted to literature and to the silence that is appropriate to it.' Chronic ill health forced Blanchot to retreat from public life when he was still young (he made a brief return during the events of May 1968); from then on, most of his relationships would be maintained by letter so that even his closest friendships were not untouched by literature.

Blanchot tirelessly draws a connection between anxiety and writing, yet in contrast to the muscular angst of his contemporaries Sartre and Camus, he does not fail to describe everything that weighs lightly on the anxious writer. In 'From Anguish to Language' (as translated by Charlotte Mandell), Blanchot writes:

> The writer finds himself in the increasingly comic condition of having nothing to write, of having no means with which to write it, and of being constrained by the utter necessity of always writing it … It seems wretched and preposterous that anguish, which opens and closes the heavens, needs, in order to manifest itself, the activity of a man sat at his table tracing letters on pieces of paper.

Blanchot draws our attention to the 'fundamental duplicity' of the literary text, the irreconcilability of its competing meanings, the way nothing is ever as it appears, every word and image seeming to demand multiple interpretations, each to the exclusion of the others. It's for this reason that Blanchot insists that reading requires 'more ignorance than knowledge,' or else 'a knowledge endowed with an immense ignorance and a gift which is not given ahead of time, which has each time to be received and acquired in forgetfulness of it, and also lost.' None of this is to deny the various forms of knowledge that can be produced 'about' a text. But it is to affirm that there is another level, which might be the most significant level, at which reading cannot produce anything at all, or nothing that is solid enough to survive the act of reading. As if the truths sought by reading were destined to dissolve under the very light that makes them visible.

I first started reading Blanchot's essays around the time that the headache started, and since then, he has been the author who, more than any other, I have found myself rereading – an experience that, from a certain perspective, has been remarkably unprofitable in that it has failed to bring about the familiarity that one might expect. It is the strangest thing. Each time I read Blanchot I enjoy the feeling of understanding, or of approaching an understanding that is just ever-so-slightly in front of me, yet whenever I get to the end of an essay, or a page, or often a single paragraph, I find myself completely unable to summarize what I have just read. Far from being a process of familiarization and assimilation, my years of rereading of Blanchot have been more like a ceaseless process of forgetting occasionally broken by flashes of understanding.

Perhaps this is as it should be. According to Roland Barthes, rereading is paradoxically the very thing that 'saves the text from repetition.' Repetition is the logic of the market, in which everything is fully legible, every Y the new X. Where those who never reread are destined to 'to read the same story everywhere' – to repeatedly find sameness in difference – rereading affirms the difference in sameness, the non-identity of every text with itself. Rereading, Barthes suggests, does not exchange the text for its true interpretation; what it reveals, he writes, is not 'the *real* text, but a plural text: the same and new.' Barthes's Heraclitan celebration of rereading might add a different emphasis to Beckett's gesture of rereading his own story. If rereading ultimately estranges a text from itself, multiplying its non-identity and novelty, then understanding a text may require us to give up our fantasies of understanding it completely.

TRANSPARENCY

'What could I say to reassure you?' the doctor asked me one day. By now it had been more than a year since I had first visited her office. I could sense the frustration in her voice, and in a way, I sympathized with her. If I'd been able to answer, I had no doubt she would have said the magic words.

In *The Birth of the Clinic*, Michel Foucault dates the 'great break' in modern diagnostics to the day when the anatomist Marie Francois Xavier Bichat, addressing a group of physicians in 1801, said that 'for twenty years, from morning to night, you have taken notes at patients' bedsides' – adding, and not without a touch of impatience, that all these efforts, all this talk, had only yielded 'a succession of incoherent phenomena.' 'Open up a few corpses,' he declared, and 'you will dissipate at once the darkness that observation alone could not.'

Some months earlier Bichat had been appointed to the old Hôtel-Dieu, the venerable Paris institution whose long, grey facades (rebuilt at midcentury during Haussmann's renovation) would haunt Rilke's first impressions of the city one hundred years later, reminding him that 'in this vast city there are legions of the sick, armies of the dying, whole populations of the dead.'

It has been said that in his first six months in this necropolis Bichat had opened six hundred corpses. Although the exact circumstances of his own death the following year remain uncertain, he seems to have fallen down the hospital stairs. According to certain accounts, Bichat's quest for knowledge was punished in the style of a Greek myth when he contracted typhoid from an unsealed corpse so that it was in a fevered state that he made the fateful fall. By that time, however, Bichat had reoriented medicine away from the observation of subjective symptoms to the pathological lesion: hidden but always in principle legible. In Foucault's words, by 'plunging from the manifest to the hidden,' Bichat had left the world with a new way of 'reading' the insides of bodies, thus making way for the modern 'medical gaze.'

Two centuries on, I longed to subject myself to that gaze: to have my flesh rendered transparent, its secrets laid bare. I was fortunate enough to have been born into an age when it has become possible to see inside bodies without even needing to break the skin. It would be hard to overstate how incredible that is. For the longest time, man's interior remained separated from his experience of himself by a veil that he knew never to cross on pain of injury and death. Beneath that veil it led an autonomous existence whose occasional stirrings could be felt but not seen, and never really understood.

In the final years of the nineteenth century, technologies started to emerge that could finally dissipate this darkness, illuminating the causes behind countless medical conditions. In 1895, the German physicist Wilhelm Röntgen discovered X-rays (the 'X' was to denote 'unknown'). By 1910 X-ray machines were common diagnostic tools in hospitals and at tuberculosis sanatoria, where they assisted in the early detection of tubercular lesions by complementing, and increasingly usurping, older tools and techniques.

Across the twentieth century, X-rays would be joined by MRI, ultrasound, CT, and PET scans – technologies that have transformed medical diagnosis while giving a new focus to the hypochondriac fantasy of knowing the body. 'I observe the physician with the same diligence as he the disease,' wrote Donne in the seventeenth century. Today, I suspect the doctor is less often the object of such fantasies than an obstacle to them – a gatekeeper of the medical knowledge that is promised by technology. *The Magic Mountain* charts this transition. In it the doctor's stethoscope provides 'only the acoustic indications; real diagnostic certainty we shall only arrive at when … the X-ray and photography have taken place. Then,' Hans says, and only then, 'we shall have positive knowledge.'

*

Dreams of complete transparency have long haunted the hypochondriac imagination. 'While a watch is up in its case,' writes James Boswell in 'On Hypochondria,' 'we cannot see how the operations of its curious machinery are carried on.' If only, he goes on, 'our bodies were transparent, so that we could see one anothers [sic] sentiments and passions working as we see bees in a glass-hive.'

Boswell's wish is perhaps the meaning behind one of the stranger fancies recorded by Robert Burton in *The Anatomy of Melancholy*: the so-called 'glass delusion' that swept early-modern Europe. Glass men first began to appear in medieval Europe. The first recorded case of somebody believing their entire body to have been transformed was Charles VI of France, in the late fourteenth century. Similar cases begin to proliferate in the sixteenth century, as glassmaking techniques increasingly left their Venetian stronghold to spread across western Europe. Technical developments meant that glass became a material that was increasingly available to outfit the windows, spectacles, dinnerware, and delusions of ever-larger swaths of the population. By 1712, when Alexander Pope came to write 'The Rape of the Lock,' it was possible to read of 'maids turn'd bottles, [who] call aloud for corks.'

What fantasy could better speak to the tenuousness of the self, the fragile border separating outside and in? Charles VI is said to have swaddled himself in blankets to prevent his buttocks from shattering. Writing in 1600 Simon Goulart tells us that such patients 'flee all company for fear of being broken.' In 1607 Thomas Walkington wrote of a 'ridiculous foole, of Venice, [who] verily thought his shoulders and buttockes were made of britle glasse; wherefore he ... never durst sitte downe to meat, lest he should have broken his crackling hinderparts.'

In Descartes's *Meditations* the glass man represents the furthest reaches of madness, as well as a dark (if disavowed) reflection of the philosopher himself. In the early-modern European imagination, the glass man became a well-known trope, a sort of shorthand for hypochondriac melancholy in its severest and most extravagant form.

The glass delusion is best memorialized by Cervantes's 'The Glass Graduate.' Published in 1613, eight years before the first edition of Burton's *Anatomy*, Cervantes's novella concerns the unhappy fate of Thomas Rodaja, a young foundling-cum-law-student who succumbs to the delusion after eating a bewitched quince. A physician cures his physical malady but is unable to 'remove that of the mind; so that when he was at last pronounced cured, he was still afflicted with the strangest madness ... The unhappy man imagined that he was entirely made of glass.'

Under the spell of this delusion, Rodaja begins performing a series of prophylactic rituals that appear to be both attempts to mitigate his illness and ways of expressing it. He walks in the middle of the street lest a roof tile should fall on his head and break it. In the winter he takes lodgings and buries himself to the neck in straw. In the summer he sleeps outdoors. He requests a 'case' in which to 'enclose the brittle vase of his body,' and, like a holy man, starts going about Salamanca barefoot in surplice and cloth.

But the most surprising aspect of this strange tale is that Rodaja's glassy condition seems to have many benefits. He puns, he exposes pretensions, and he can discourse eloquently on seemingly any topic. After all, he explains, no longer made 'of flesh and bones,' it is to be expected that he should be able to converse 'with all the more effect ... since glass, being a substance of more delicate subtlety, permits the soul to act with more promptitude and efficacy than it can be expected to do in the heavier body formed of mere earth.' Thus with Cervantes's story we have an early-modern version of a fantasy that, I am tempted to say, continues to sit behind our dreams of transparency: a mind that has been released from its servitude to an opaque and lumbering physical self.

Glass men began to disappear in the eighteenth century, perhaps as glass, increasingly commonplace, ceased to provide a suitable vessel for our hopes about the body. But the dream persists, now directed toward newer technologies such as the full-body MRI scans currently being offered by many private companies. The glass body represents the hypochondriac's gravest fears and their most extravagant fantasies: it is the dream of a body that is fragile and vulnerable but also fully and finally knowable.

*

Transparency is one of the cardinal virtues of neoliberal society, not only when it comes to health, but also in the realms of politics, technology, and interpersonal relationships. In a characteristically wide-ranging and bombastic polemic called *The Transparency Society*, Byung-Chul Han argues that the contemporary equation of transparency with trustworthiness can only occur 'in a society where the meaning of "trust" has been massively compromised.'

In *The Phenomenology of Illness*, the philosopher Havi Carel describes the way illness can break the 'existential feeling of trust' underlying the healthy individual's ordinary relationship to their body, a phenomenon she calls 'the loss of bodily transparency.' When this happens the body ceases to be the locus of identity and expression and becomes something closer to the Cartesian body, a foreign entity whose sensations are suspect. Trust requires a pact with uncertainty, a suspension of the will to know. Meanwhile, as Han writes, transparency, raised to an absolute value, quickly gives way to practices of 'total control and surveillance.'

The opposite of transparency is opacity; more figuratively, it is blindness, the culmination of Oedipus's attempts to uncover the truth about himself. In 'On Arrogance' Wilfred Bion rereads the founding myth of psychoanalysis and argues that this is the tale's true cautionary meaning. Contrary to Freud's interpretation, he argues, incest is in fact only an ancillary offence in a story in which a much graver crime is punished: the 'arrogance of Oedipus in vowing to lay bare the truth at no matter what cost.' For certain patients, writes Bion, it is the dream of possessing the complete truth (not the mother) that dominates their psychic life. In meeting with such cases, he warns, the analyst must be very careful to avoid becoming an 'accessory' as the analytic space itself becomes saturated with this epistemological fantasy.

From the time that he and Josef Breuer published *Studies in Hysteria* in 1895 – the same year that Röntgen attached the prefix 'X' to his newly discovered rays – Freud was given to voicing dreams of complete transparency when speaking about his new science. Most famously in the oft-quoted line: 'Where the Id was, there the Ego shall be,' more clearly expressed without his translator James Strachey's Latin: 'Where it was, there I will be.' As if to arrogantly suggest that, by way of his new method, the dark regions of the unconscious mind would finally dissipate in the of light self-understanding.

Yet it was Freud's great innovation to see that everything could be read – and therefore reread. This was even true of dreams, which most people before Freud had considered to be nothing, or nothing important. In *The Interpretation of Dreams*, Freud pauses a discussion of Hamlet, another interminable rereader, to note that, like 'all genuinely creative writings,' dreams and neurotic symptoms are 'capable of being "overinterpreted" and indeed need to be, if they are to be fully understood.' With these words, Freud is suggesting that understanding a text fully means understanding that no understanding of it will ever be full; that no reading can be complete that does not leave space for other readings.

Later in that book, in a section fittingly titled 'The Forgetting of Dreams,' Freud writes of 'a passage in even the most thoroughly interpreted dream which has to be left obscure.' In every interpretation, he writes, one will eventually come upon 'a tangle of dream-thoughts which cannot be unravelled and which moreover adds nothing to our knowledge of the content of the dream. This is the dream's navel, the spot where it reaches into the unknown.' The blindness that Freud is writing about here is not a divine punishment. He is writing of knowledge being greeted, in a friendly way, with discreet smiles and the tipping of hats, by its other. If unknowing is the ultimate destination of all attempts to know one's own unconscious, then the aim of psychoanalysis perhaps consists in only this:

accommodating the patient to the incontrovertible fact of their opacity to themselves.

*

A little over a year after the headache began, the doctor referred me to a specialist. A few months later I visited the Royal Sussex County Hospital, where the neurologist listened to me speak, nodded sympathetically, and then ordered an MRI. A few weeks later, I had the scan. A fortnight after that, a letter arrived. In its entirety, it read: 'Dear Mr Rees, Your brain is reported as normal.' No follow-up appointment, no onward referral, just a signature at the bottom of the page that I could not read. I still have that letter somewhere. For the rest of the day, I floated about in a state of restless euphoria, feeling as if my feet had left the ground. For some time after that, I didn't think much about the headache, or about my health.

Up late one night some months later, I found myself looking into error rates within radiology – I can't remember the train of thought that led me there. On average, it's around 3 to 5 percent. This was not that bad, I thought, at least not as bad as I had feared. Then I googled the number of annual radiology scans in the UK; that year it was around 40 million. If 4 percent of those were wrong, this amounted to 1.6 million incorrect scans, a number that was certainly big enough to include me. Actually, this was only in day-to-day general practice where mostly normal images are being viewed. Among those who go on to be diagnosed with significant illness, the rate is higher, more like 30 percent. Which is to say, if one does have a tumour, it's not uncommon for it to be missed, whether by the scan itself or, more commonly, by the radiologist who reads it. In a study of those diagnosed with a lung carcinoma, I eventually learned, the lesion could retrospectively be found in 90 percent of 'negative' scans.

The novelist Lynne Tillman writes about her shock when, between four doctors, there were three different interpretations of her mother's brain scan: 'No certainty in reading the brain and, like reading any text, an MRI requires interpretation.' Most lesions missed by radiologists are in the first or last images in a series, those that might be passed over more quickly as they scan through. For some reason learning this fact disturbed me more than the numbers themselves, perhaps because I could picture myself flicking like that through a book, my mind elsewhere. For nearly two years I'd wanted nothing more than a negative scan result. The letter in hand, now all I could think about was my tumour, a mark on the page, missed by the person who had read it. There was, I was beginning to realize, no way to get around interpretation.

PLAYING THE HYPOCHONDRIAC

By the summer of 1913, it had been nearly a year since Kafka and Felice Bauer had begun corresponding, and several months since they'd started speaking of marriage, speculatively at first, hypothetically, but at some point those weightless words had solidified into a commitment and then, worse still, a plan. For Kafka, this initiated a period of crisis. He truly did want to marry Felice. The problem was that he also wanted not to marry her, and that these two possibilities were incompatible. For as long as his desires had been private, their incommensurability could be contained. Now, ambivalence spilled over into panic.

Kafka concocted a plan. He couldn't break his commitment, that was impossible, but by eliciting a refusal from a paternal authority he could ensure the marriage would never come to pass. There were two options. If his own father forbade it, it would be a humiliation; he'd die of shame or else be left with no other option: he would have to march straight to Berlin and marry Felice in defiance. So, instead Kafka set about convincing Herr Bauer to refuse him, a more appealing prospect that could later on be spun into an amusing or even flattering coffee house tale.

On the morning of 21 August, Kafka visited his local bookseller, from whom he acquired the works of Kierkegaard. Kafka approvingly read the Danish philosopher, drawing inspiration from his missives and evasions, his broken engagement and cultivated misery. Then he sat down at his desk. 'Dear Herr Bauer,' he began; and, after a few pleasantries, a confession: 'I have deluded your daughter with my letters.' But immediately following that, a series of equivocations: 'as a rule, I have not meant to deceive her,' he says, 'although sometimes I have … I really don't know.' Kafka then proceeds to list the character flaws that made him unappealing as a potential son-in-law: 'I am taciturn, unsociable, morose, selfish, a hypochondriac, and actually in poor health.'

'Well,' he concludes his letter to Felice's father, unconsciously evoking his breakthrough story of a year earlier, 'You be the judge!'

*

What does it mean to confess, 'I am a hypochondriac'? Surely the utterance is a performative contradiction: a true hypochondriac doesn't say they're a hypochondriac, they simply say they have cancer or Lyme disease. Or else, like Tony Hancock, they say that hypochondria is the one illness they don't have. To say that I am a hypochondriac, meanwhile, is to say I believe I have, for instance, stage-four brain cancer, while also saying I don't believe I have it, or that I don't believe my belief that I have it. What does it mean to say that about oneself?

Confessing to being a hypochondriac is like the philosophical paradox that asks whether one can truthfully declare oneself to be a liar. Which is probably why, for the most part, we are better at diagnosing hypochondria in other people than in ourselves: you are a hypochondriac, I have well-founded concerns. And yet online support groups are full of entries from self-diagnosed sufferers of health anxiety: people whose problem, like Kafka's, is that they don't fully believe they have a problem.

In the 1920s a German psychiatrist wrote about a patient who suffered from the painful hypochondriacal fixation that he might have hypochondria, a fear that, if 'true,' means the patient would cease to be a hypochondriac (therefore becoming one). Not simply a logical parlour game, the paradox speaks to what is one of the most distinctive features of hypochondriac doubt, its recursiveness, its tendency to constantly call itself into question, to cross out its own name.

Kafka's diaries and letters abound with self-immolating doubts ('I have not meant to deceive her … although sometimes I have … I really don't know'), so it is perhaps not surprising that he seems to have discerned all this, the way any confession of hypochondria seems to evaporate in transit. His solution was practical: he was, as he said, a hypochondriac – and he was actually in poor health. I suspect this double consciousness is not at all uncommon. For my part, I had little difficulty in seeing that friends had a point when they suggested that my worries were hypochondriacal. In fact I accepted it, invited it. The label, after all, was hardly without its consolations, and these more than compensated for any embarrassment it conferred (in the inflated terminology of official psychiatry, 'stigmatization'). 'Yes,' I got in the habit of saying, 'I am a hypochondriac.' An absurd, hopeless hypochondriac.

Psychiatry calls this 'insight': the patient's capacity to recognize they may be suffering from a mental illness. And yet my capacity, or desire, to accept that I was a hypochondriac did nothing to loosen the grip my fears had over me, the conviction with which I held them to be true. I simply held opposing views on the status of my health, reasoning that a hypochondriac can also become sick – and of course sooner or later, most of them will – and that I happened to be both. What was more, by one of those remarkable ironies to which every person believes that they alone are susceptible, the identity of my actual illness happened to coincide with the one that I'd imagined.

*

It was at this time that I started compulsively watching films and TV shows about hypochondriacs, even those, like the films of Woody Allen, that I otherwise felt to be of dubious quality. 'Oh, God, there's a tumor in my head the size of a basketball!' Allen says to himself in *Hannah and her Sisters*. I also found myself identifying with the feline protagonist of *The Hypo-Chondri-Cat*, Warner Brothers' undeniably minor animated entertainment in which an anxious cat suffers at the hands of two trickster mice.

I had a special fondness for *Seinfeld*'s George Costanza. In a famous scene, George clutches his chest in the diner and yells: 'I think I'm having a heart attack!' Elaine and Jerry roll their eyes, and we can't help but sympathise with George's long-suffering friends.

This type of comedy rests on dramatic irony, on the distance between how the hypochondriac sees themself and how we know things truly stand. That is why it is so reassuring: the absurd characters it depicts are protected by the constraints of genre, as if hypochondria compensated its sufferers for their imaginary ailments by making them invulnerable to any actual disease.

We learn something about hypochondriacs, or our perceptions of them, by observing that they feature most frequently in those comic genres that favour formula and repetition: the silent comedy, the sitcom. Meanwhile, in the nineteenth-century novel, the hypochondriac is always one of those single-trait secondary characters who will not undergo any psychological evolution: at the end of the third act, the hypochondriac father or uncle will remain his tiresome old self in a world that has been transformed around him.

Why are these characters funny? For Henri Bergson, comedy reveals the 'mechanical encrusted on the living,' and there does seem to be something mechanistic about the hypochondriac's serially repeated fears: slipping endlessly upon the banana skin of his fixation, the hypochondriac is comically incapable of learning from past mistakes. It is this tendency to repeat that leads Brian Dillon to suggest that the hypochondriac resembles the clown, and it's true that many comedians have cultivated hypochondria as part of their schtick. But the hypochondriac also resembles the clown's sidekick and comedic foil, the straight man. Where the clown is charmingly eccentric, the straight man is deadly serious. He is humourless, which is precisely what makes him so funny, since, as Lauren Berlant has observed, whoever is not in on a joke can easily become the joke.

According to Berlant, humourlessness 'involves the encounter with a fundamental intractability in oneself or in others' that results from 'someone's insistence that their version of a situation should rule the relational dynamic.' Humourlessness occurs when a person bristles to find that their sovereignty – their 'fantasy of self-ratifying control over a situation or space' – has been cast scandalously into question by the dissenting view of another. Humourlessness is therefore a kind of failure of relation, an individual's inability to consider – to humour – their interlocutor's alternative perspective on themselves, the world, or the situation; as when, in response to Jerry and Elaine's doubts that he is in a state of cardiac arrest, George responds as though his sovereignty is what has been called into question: 'Why can't I have a heart attack? I'm allowed!'

Berlant goes on to list the hypochondriac among the denizens of the humourless, and indeed there are times, particularly when in the grips of a fixation, when the hypochondriac is a rather humourless character, times of intense anxiety when the hypochondriac identifies fully with their beliefs and any disbelief, any want of seriousness or sympathy on the part of a listener, can only be met with indignation. I had a friend like that, although he tended to burn bridges, since the advice that he solicited could only be received as an attack. Friends were invited to condemn the wavering convictions of other friends as to the reality of the dread disease, and when this condemnation failed to reach the required pitch of outrage they, too, were dropped.

But I suspect that for the most part hypochondriacs occupy a more ambiguous vantage on their own suffering. According to the psychiatrist Arthur Kleinman, 'It is ironic that hypochondriacs, faced with medical disbelief, are forced to act as though they lacked irony.' In reality, argues Kleinman, there are very few patients who 'take the body overly seriously, humorlessly.' Most hypochondriacs, to borrow Anne Boyer's phrase, are also reverse hypochondriacs. Uncommon are those with George Costanza's inflexible, unreflexive self-certainty, since, unlike their fictional counterparts, real-life hypochondriacs have generally been granted some insight into their condition, and, moreover, are likely to have learned the risks of appearing humourless.

'How fatally the entire want of humour cripples the mind,' wrote Alice James in the diary in which she also recorded the symptoms of her nervous ailments. 'What an awful loss it is that we can't see our own follies, they must be so much more exquisite than any one's else.' As James goes on to suggest, the problem with humourlessness is that it is very funny (revealing, as Bergson would put it, 'a certain mechanical inelasticity' embedded in the personality). The more one insists on being taken seriously, the more irresistibly one extends the invitation for people to do the exact opposite, like the child in the throes of a tantrum who demands that the adults stop laughing at them immediately.

Which is to say that the hypochondriac, who after all wishes to be believed, and therefore to be taken seriously, would do well to avoid seeming too inflexibly attached to their beliefs. If they wish to avoid appearing humourless – and therefore absurd, ridiculous, an unreliable narrator – hypochondriacs need to be urbane about the possibility that they're wrong. Surely this is why hypochondriacs joke so much, which is not to say that all of them are funny. But in order to appear credible, a hypochondriac must learn to ironize their own fears; must learn to say, 'I am a hypochondriac.'

And yet they must also take care to go on believing themselves, not permitting themselves to be diverted from the urgent task of seeking medical care. As Kierkegaard warns in *Either/Or*, clownishness can be as much of a rhetorical straitjacket as humourlessness:

> A fire broke out backstage in a theatre. The clown came out to warn the public; they thought it was a joke and applauded. He repeated it; the acclaim was even greater. I think that's just how the world will come to an end: to the general applause from wits who believe it's a joke.

At once straight man and clown, a hypochondriac must take themself seriously while suspecting themself to be a joke.

*

Although in his letters Kafka constantly calls himself a hypochondriac, he almost never does so in his journal. It is as if the performance of hypochondria requires an audience.

With doctors I often felt the need to overperform my conviction that I was physically sick. In truth, nothing was less certain, since I knew, or thought I knew, or hoped, that the symptoms I was experiencing could be merely tricks wrought upon my body by my anxious mind. And yet I also knew that giving free expression to these thoughts would be inviting the doctor to funnel me down a mental health pathway, whose endpoint, I feared, would be a few sessions of cognitive behavioural therapy. I imagined myself in a windowless room, listening to epidemiological data intended to disabuse me of my maladaptive thoughts. It wasn't that I thought such therapy would be ineffective. Actually, I was worried it would work – that a few words of stern reassurance from a finitely patient NHS therapist would succeed in converting concern into complacency.

When speaking to doctors, therefore, I often avoided disclosing my doubts as to the organic reality of these symptoms. And yet, any person who overplays that role starts to seem like they really might be mad. The ICD-11 rates the severity of hypochondriasis according to the level of insight ('good,' 'fair,' 'poor,' and 'absent'), with the patients at the lower end of this spectrum appearing 'delusional in the degree of conviction.' Those rare patients entirely lacking in insight or irony – patients whose humourless assessment of their situation permits of no alternative readings – can be diagnosed with 'monosymptomatic hypochondriacal psychosis.' Sanity, so as not to appear psychotic, needs to be a little urbane with regard to its own limits.

So when it was put to me by the doctor that my headaches might be perpetuated by the tension caused by my worrying over their potential cause, I knowingly assented to the interpretation. Yes, I agreed, that was possible. It was true that these headaches had left me a little worried of late. Maybe this was making things worse? Of course, there was subterfuge in my candour. By dispassionately accepting the possibility of a psychosomatic explanation, I was asking the doctor to behold a mind that had no need to somatize; performing the role of a person so well-adjusted that, should he be feeling unwell, there must be something really the matter with him.

This being said, in other areas of my life, I found myself wholeheartedly playing into and up to the role of hypochondriac. Playing the hypochondriac ensured that no one could accuse me of humourless devotion to my delusions, blindness to my own blind spots. There is space within even the most straitened role provided one has chosen it. I chose to be a hypochondriac, which is not to say I pretended to be one. But I consented to it, conspired with it. I hammered things up and overacted. I made myself foolish in the eyes of others, inviting friends to ridicule my fears and thereby reduce them to more liveable proportions.

I learnt to ironize myself; I became my own satirist. I started referring drolly and in passing to diseases whose names carried an almost supernatural power, and in this way sought to lessen the sway they held over me; the profound, bodily response their mere mention could instill in me; the superstitious and fatalistic trains of thought that were set in motion by seeing their names mentioned in print. This was a power grab; it was an attempt to transform fear into eccentricity. In *Annie Hall* there is a scene where Allen's character is asked if he is being serious or if, on the contrary, he is joking. God, what a terrible question, I remember thinking. No one should have to answer that. When I received the MRI results telling me 'your brain is normal,' I wrote A+ and stuck it on the refrigerator. I proudly showed it to visitors.

By ironizing my fears, I was able to stop myself from going under. I was able to keep my passport for the kingdom of the well. The performance was not seamless, however. It tended to come apart at night. Lying in bed it would occur to me that whatever was going to happen to me, it would only be my fault: I knew I was sick yet was allowing myself to be seduced by the fantasy that I was imagining it, that I was, as friends insisted and I too eagerly agreed, 'a hypochondriac.'

But on the whole, by learning to say 'I am a hypochondriac' I was able to hold things together. In popular imagination the hypochondriac is a comic character who, always imagining himself or herself to be sick, is, in reality, healthy. I set about playing this role with studied irrationality, never missing an opportunity to clownishly perform anxieties which previously I'd only felt. There was in this an element of my timeworn defensive posturing, a determination to be in on the joke if I was going to be it. But I can see now that this was also an exercise in magical thinking. If I could convincingly play the hypochondriac, then I wouldn't – could not – actually be sick.

The most celebrated comic hypochondriac is surely Argan, the protagonist of the 1673 comic farce *Le malade imaginaire* by Molière (the stage name of Jean-Baptiste Poquelin). Molière's play does not actually use the word 'hypochondria,' and yet for centuries English-language productions have often been staged under the title *The Hypochondriac*, the name that was given to the play in 1714 by its first English translator, John Ozell.

Argan is a wealthy, invalided widower who is forever coughing and complaining and cataloguing his symptoms, although he tends to get prickly when he is asked about the identity of his illness. Argan's fantasies have been nursed by his physician and apothecarist, for whom he provides a stable source of income. The plot of Molière's comedy involves Argan attempting to marry his daughter to an unappealing young physician, with the aim of defraying his medical costs. When she refuses, Argan threatens to put her in a convent, and his brother and servant work to prevent the unjust punishment from coming to pass. Meanwhile Argan's acquisitive new wife, suspecting that his 'illness' will fail to yield the bequeathment for which she has married him, schemes to swindle the lovesick old man out of his riches.

Above all it is Argan's humourlessness that makes him an easy target for those who wish to exploit his many blind spots. Argan is convinced that he is adored by his wife and revered as the head of his family, when in reality these rigid and idealizing beliefs mean that he can be efficiently gamed by every character in the play, his servant included, since one need only pamper his preferred self-image in order to get what one wants. Of course, Argan's humourlessness is exploited most ruthlessly of all by Molière, who invites his audience to share in the joke of a man, a hypochondriac, who, overserious and possessing absolutely no insight into his own condition, is comically deluded in every single aspect of his life.

Molière's play culminates with the comic genre's obligatory happy ending. By playing dead, Argan is able to see what everyone really thinks of him. Soon, his avaricious wife is exposed; his daughter is permitted to marry her preferred suitor; and Argan himself is 'cured' after being persuaded to become a doctor himself. This last development turns out to require no special training, since medical knowledge, according to Molière's play, amounts to almost nothing at all. Doctors know the Greek and Latin names of countless diseases and have learned to speak very highly of their own abilities. But in reality they haven't the faintest idea how to cure the sick. In fact, doctors are the mirror image of hypochondriacs: both discourse eloquently upon disease in flighty abstraction from the actual body. United in a single person, the inflated confidence of the one will abolish the anxieties of the other.

This view on medicine is also taken up in Molière's *Monsieur de Pourceaugnac*, a comic opera that appears to be a preparatory sketch for the rightly more famous play. The medical satire is even more bracing in this earlier play, in which physicians not only fail to cure diseases but go so far as to inflict them on their patients through the act of diagnosis: 'I enjoin both you and your daughter not to celebrate the wedding without my consent, upon pain of ... undergoing all the diseases which we choose to lay upon you.' Monsieur de Pourceaugnac, a dull, poorly dressed provincial, arrives in Paris to marry Julia. Her affections lie elsewhere – the marriage has been arranged by her father – and so to thwart things Julia's friends play a series a tricks on the unsuspecting Pourceaugnac, including an elaborate ruse that sees him diagnosed with hypochondria:

[O]ur patient here present is unhappily attacked, affected, possessed, and disordered by that kind of madness which we properly name hypochondriac melancholy; a very trying kind of madness… In proof of what I say, and as an incontestable diagnostic of it, you need only consider that great seriousness, that sadness, accompanied by signs of fearfulness and suspicion[.]

After conferring with his colleague, the physician decides that Pourceaugnac 'should be freely phlebotomized; by which I mean that there should be frequent and abundant bleedings … and, at the same time, that he should be purged, deobstructed, and evacuated by fit and suitable purgatives.' Diseases might often be imaginary, but, warns Molière, the often harmful cures proposed by unscrupulous doctors are very real indeed.

With *Le malade imaginaire*, Molière gives us a different notion of cure. The comedy ends with Argan's farcical graduation ceremony, held in nonsense Latin – a rowdy, carnivalesque celebration of folly in its different guises. In this final scene, Argan has finally learned how to play; he has been transformed from straight man into clown. It is a lovely ending: Argan's maladaptive fears have not been cured through disillusionment. Instead, the other characters have created ways to enable Argan to live more expansively within the confines of his fantasy. It is the beautiful and unglamorous suggestion of Molière's play that this may well be the kindest thing that we can do for one another.

For Molière, the condition and its cure both exist at the level of imagination, which this scene suggests is also the level of performance, of theatre – what, in *The Tempest*, Prospero calls an 'insubstantial pageant.' With this final scene, Molière's play becomes something more than a comic debunking, the withdrawal of masks. Rather, it proposes that the cure for hypochondria resides in the search for a better, the more enchanting, illusion. I wonder what it would mean to take this recommendation seriously. A certain type of psychological therapy seeks to placate those who fret about their health by apprising them of, and thus adapting them to, 'the facts.' Another approach might be to meet the knowledge-seeking hypochondriac where they find themselves, and to help them make a home in the hazier regions of enchantment, and nescience, and uncertainty. Not in the name of wilful ignorance, but simply of a more various orientation toward life where the compulsion to know no longer rules supreme.

*

Thinking of the final scene of Molière's play, I'm reminded of William Hazlitt. In the winter of 1815, he saw a performance by some visiting South Asian jugglers at a theatre near the Strand, a spectacle whose transporting effect on him was undiminished when he came to describe it six years later in 'The Indian Jugglers.' According to Hazlitt, the jugglers' mastery is undeniable: 'A single error of a hair's-breadth, of the smallest conceivable portion of time, would be fatal: the precision of the movements must be like a mathematical truth, their rapidity is like lightning.' And yet all this effort – for what? Regarding the jugglers, Hazlitt asks: 'Is it then a trifling power we see at work, or is it not something next to miraculous?'

In the literary high-wire that follows, Hazlitt leans one way and then the other, unable, or perhaps unwilling, to decide once and for all. At the outset, he is mirthful and buoyant: 'Man, thou art a wonderful animal, and thy ways past finding out! Thou canst do strange things, but thou turnest them to little account!' His levity wanes, however, when he wonders what separates his own art from the pursuit of this inconsequential perfection. Before long, disquiet gives way to darker thoughts: 'I ask what there is that I can do as well as this? Nothing. What have I been doing all my life?' he wonders. 'Have I passed my time in pouring words like water into empty sieves?'

Kafka, too, seemed to find a super-egoic reflection of himself in the circus or the sideshow performer. Most famously his hunger artist, who starves himself to the intrigue then boredom of the public, though in the end, only because he has been unable to find any palatable food. And the trapeze artist of the near-contemporaneous 'First Sorrow,' who has mastered 'his art in all its perfection,' and who refuses, between acts, to set foot on earth. Kafka is troubled by the way his circus performers sacrifice everything to what might really amount to nothing – to a groundless pursuit of perfection. Isn't that what he was doing, too, staying up all night, inventing situations, tracing letters on pieces of paper? An absurd fate: 'what frail or even nonexistent ground I live on,' he wrote to Max Brod, 'over a darkness from which the dark power emerges … [and] destroys my life. Writing sustains me, but isn't it more accurate to say that it sustains this kind of life?'

For Kafka the absurdity of writing was intimately connected with hypochondria: two baseless yet all-consuming enterprises that bordered on the ghostly. In one of his earliest letters to Felice, he told her of his 'self-enamored hypochondria,' a confession that came in response to Felice's request that he exercise more 'moderation and purpose' with his writing. Kafka's rather humourless reply:

Shouldn't I stake everything I have on the one spot where I have a firm footing? If I did not do so, what a hopeless fool I would be! It is possible that my writing is nothing, but in that case it is quite certain, beyond any doubt, that I am absolutely nothing. If I spare myself in this respect, then properly speaking I am not really sparing myself, but killing myself.

For his part Hazlitt will seek to overcome these thoughts by suggesting, in fairly conventional terms, that the 'bungling' of the literary artist may ultimately be of higher value than the jugglers' mere perfection. And yet, seemingly in spite of himself, he keeps bringing the jugglers back up. It's as if, six years on, he still can't stop returning to the scene of that performance, a scene whose pleasure won't be dispelled via any high-minded aesthetics. In the end, the essay becomes a celebration, written 'between jest and earnest,' of an array of popular performers: jugglers, sword swallowers, the legendary Sadler's Wells rope dancer Richer, and the fives player John Cavanagh.

For Hazlitt the essay form, iterative and multivocal, provides an arena for these mixed feelings, this uncertainty that would be deadly to the juggler's art. In 'The Essay as Form,' Adorno would argue something similar: 'Luck and play are essential to it,' he writes, suggesting that, far from being to its detriment, it is in fact one of the essay's virtues that its 'interpretations are not philologically definitive and conscientious; in principle they are over-interpretations.' In contrast, say, to the academic monograph, the essay does not deign to exhaust its topic; it leaves space. Likewise, in the first of his Hypochondriack essays, Boswell discusses the advantages of the apparently slight personal essay over more definitive works, declaring that the 'periodical paper of instruction and entertainment may be reckoned one of the happiest inventions of modern times.'

Despite seeming, on first appearances, like a brooding reckoning with art's proximity to amusement, 'The Indian Jugglers' becomes something altogether more interesting: a celebration of insubstantial pageantry in its different guises, including above all that of the essay itself. We are a long way here from Kafka. Its own kind of performance, Hazlitt's essay embraces the possibilities opened up by suspending the impulse to distinguish between instruction and entertainment, jest and earnest, the trifling and the miraculous. As if to be caught up in the enthusiasm of performance allows for a pleasurable, if temporary, loosening of the demand to answer what might really be a very tedious question: does it matter?

*

I didn't see a production of *Le malade imaginaire* during those years in which I resembled Argan. By that time, I'd abandoned my own desire to pursue a medical career, so one treatment pathway had been closed to me. Nevertheless, had I seen *Le malade* during those years I suspect its effect on me would have been consoling. In Molière's comedy, there is never any question of whether, beneath the pageantry and illusion, Argan might actually be sick. In the reassuring logic of his play, Argan cannot be sick in reality for the precise reason that he is a hypochondriac, someone who is sick within the imagination. To be sick is ruled out by definition, as though hypochondria conferred its victims with a kind of logical immunity.

This is a comic tradition which, in more recent times, has frequently been reprised. We know that George Costanza will

not really be sick precisely because of his humourless commitment to the view that he is sick. This is what makes *Seinfeld*
funny and not in the least bit alarming. It is the fantasy that
animates every desire to play the hypochondriac.

But as the hypochondriac certainly knows, even if they
permit themselves to consider it only at night as they lie in bed,
the role they are playing is not one in which it is possible to
lose themselves completely like those ethereal players in *The
Tempest* who vanish once the masque finishes. 'These our actors,'
Prospero declares, 'were all spirits, and are melted into air, into
thin air.' In reality we know that beneath airy fantasy and
performance there always remains the physical body, a body
that is susceptible to sickness and injury, and sooner or later –
and always too soon – consigned to the mortality that is its
only birth-right.

When *Le malade imaginaire* opened at the Théâtre du Palais-
Royal on 10 February 1673, the role of Argan was filled by
Molière himself, who in addition to being Paris's most revered
playwright was also one of its favourite actors. Playing Argan
does not place excessive physical demands upon an actor. For
most of the play he is either seated or recumbent, swaddled in
a blanket. He is, after all, an invalid, albeit an 'imaginary' one.
But the final scene is different altogether, full of prancing, and
parading, and prattling. Nevertheless, amid all the revelry,
Molière remained seated in his red velvet chair. It was during
this scene that on a Friday performance, one week after opening,
Molière fell into a convulsion.

Some who were in attendance that evening must surely
have been impressed by the actor's commitment to the role,
his realistic portrayal of the invalid. But the invalid was not
actually supposed to be sick. Molière composed himself. He

slipped back into the role. He was Argan again, the hypochondriac. Seeing the spluttering actor attempting to regain composure must have been alarming, a visceral reminder of the body beneath the performance, the real beneath the imaginary, the tragic that always threatens to intrude upon the comic. When the performance ended, Molière did not vanish. He returned home, and later that evening, he died of a pulmonary hemorrhage.

For some time, Molière had been following a strict milk diet, having retreated to the peaceful hamlet of Auteuil (later the birthplace of Charles Baudelaire and Marcel Proust). Molière seems to have known that he was unwell. Yet in the months leading up to his death, there was virtually no reference to his illness. Meanwhile, a friend later said that Molière had been visibly ill earlier in the day, that others had begged him not to act, but that he had insisted on the usual 4 p.m. start. Which is to say that Molière was hiding his illness, and that in playing the hypochondriac that February evening, he was playing the part of a healthy person who, in turn, plays another healthy person who believes he is sick and at one point pretends to be dead. And yet, beneath the layers of performance, and indifferent to each of these nice ironies, there was the simple, banal fact of a disease-stricken body belonging to a fifty-one-year-old man.

LATENCY

A few years ago, I was working on my serious, scholarly study of hypochondria. I had been trying so hard to be diligent but for some time things had not been going well; there was, my research was revealing to me, just so much I didn't know. One day I decided to get hold of my medical records. I suppose my academic research had reignited my curiosity. I wasn't worried, not really, I just thought it would be interesting, relevant, for the purposes of my work, to see for the first time this vast document, bursting with information, a series of manila folders stuffed with well-thumbed papers that were barely held together with elastic bands. I got in touch with my GP's practice to request the file. It felt weirdly prurient, asking for my medical records. I invented an excuse – some private provider who wanted to see it, as if there were something shameful about a desire to look myself. While I was waiting on hold I decided this was stupid and so, when I got through, just asked for it straight out. They were, after all, about me – were me, in a way, a sort of personal archive. In the end this turned out to be a routine request; I was directed toward a web form that did not ask for reasons. I wondered what it would be like, seeing it, if I would be described using any of the shibboleths supposedly used by doctors ('gomer': 'Get out of my emergency room,' etc.), if it would reactivate old fears. For several weeks, each time the doorbell rang, I anticipated the arrival of my hefty cargo. It didn't come, however, and after a while I forgot about it. Six months later I got an email, subject line: *Your medical records*. How romantic of me, I thought in retrospect, to have expected anything physical. I opened the PDF with some trepidation, and as I scrolled through the results of various routine tests, felt the weird hot pang of reading about myself in the third person, which Blanchot describes as a kind of death, before realizing they only went back two years: the time I had been registered at my current GP's practice. I called up and told this to the receptionist, who said they could try to locate older records, though this might take a long time, or else may prove impossible, generally speaking it did, especially given I had, as I'd told her, moved house almost every year for more than a decade. She asked if I'd like them to try. Yes I would, I said, quite surprised by the officiousness of my tone. Of course, the records never materialized. Perhaps they no longer exist, though I like to think they'll turn up sooner or later.

*

In *After 1945: Latency as Origin of the Present*, the critic Hans Ulrich Gumbrecht argues that, since the second half of the twentieth century, latency has come to define the collective atmosphere. Gumbrecht describes latency as a mood, a state of anxiety in which some hidden danger constantly threatens to reveal itself – but not yet. How, asks Gumbrecht, 'can we be so certain that something latent is "really there" if it eludes our very perception?' His answer is that we can't, that uncertainty is among the defining features of latency, as that which threatens to become manifest might turn out not to exist.

According to Gumbrecht, the most drastic effect of latency is to reorient one's relationship to the future: no longer a horizon of possibilities, it becomes a continual source of danger which must be kept at bay. In latency, he writes, time becomes 'frozen' as one awaits what might never arrive. It's for this reason that Gumbrecht describes latency as the opposite of emergency: where the latter suggests a 'spontaneous movement upward,' states of latency involve a 'downward movement,' the discovery of a depth from which something hidden perpetually fails to emerge.

If there is a poet laureate of states of emergency, surely it is John Donne: 'this minute I was well, and am ill, this minute,' writes Donne in the first of his *Devotions upon Emergent Occasions* of 1624, composed as he was recovering from a relapsing fever that was sweeping London. In these lines, which are among the most widely quoted in Donne's body of work, the poet describes illness as a visitation, a sudden upsurge. As an emergency.

> We study health, and we deliberate upon our meats, and drink, and air, and exercises, and we hew and we polish every stone that goes to that building; and so our health is a long and a regular work: but in a minute a cannon batters all, overthrows all, demolishes all; a sickness unprevented for our diligence, unsuspected for all our curiosity; nay, undeserved, if we consider only disorder, summons us, seizes us, possesses us, destroys us in an instant.

I first read the *Devotions* in my mid-twenties, certain I was ill but struggling to prove it. Sometime earlier my fears had gone into remission, but then they came back, newly focused around the lymph nodes in my armpits and neck. They'd been swollen for years. At some point it was obvious: hadn't this really always been where the problem lay? The brain tumour, in retrospect, was absurd, adolescent.

Real as my symptoms were, however, they were annoyingly minor, hard to distinguish from life's ordinary grievances. I was always so tired. My gums bled each time I brushed my teeth. I itched all over, and at night strange aches yawned, like whale song, through the long bones of my arms and legs.

The most profound symptom, however, was also the hardest to describe: at some deep level, sacrosanct and barely touched by doubt, I could feel there was something wrong with my blood.

It is within this context that I remember being appalled and exhilarated by this vivid description of the medical crisis. Reading Donne, I found myself secretly longing for an emergency, an event that would bring everything to the surface. I have experienced that once or twice, like the morning when, waking up in a state of anaphylaxis, I went straight to the emergency department, where I was shot with steroids that immediately brought things under control. For days I'd known something was off – scratchy throat, streaming eyes – but had been ignoring it. Now there was nothing else for it. This is the lure of emergency: a single moment that will unfreeze time, accelerate it, and release you from the state of waiting.

Rereading Donne more recently, however, it isn't only his descriptions of the medical emergency that I notice. Even as he has just been battered by fever, Donne remains haunted by states of latency. The 'greatest mischiefs,' he tells us, are those 'which are the least discerned.' Moreover, man's torment isn't that he must die, but that he must die 'by the torment of sickness; nor only that,' adds Donne, but after a life that has been 'pre-afflicted, super-afflicted with these jealousies and suspicions and apprehensions of sickness, before we can call it a sickness: we are not sure we are ill; one hand asks the other by the pulse, and our eye asks our own urine how we do.' Such fears and premonitions 'antedate the sickness,' he writes, and make it 'the more irremediable by sad apprehensions.'

Reading Donne, I'm reminded of a comment from Blanchot, who after years of suffering from disabling yet amorphous symptoms came to the conclusion that 'illness and life are one,' and that 'doctors can only give us provisional assistance in giving one the appearance of the other.' For Donne, as for Blanchot, the greatest mischief is precisely that illness does not destroy us 'in an instant.' It steals into life wearing the garb of health. So that, long before illness has finally emerged into the open, I can never quite know that I am well.

In fact, Donne will go on to suggest, the worst disease of all would be one that did not produce any symptoms at all, a disease (one is tempted to call it life itself) that performed its abominable offices in secret, never emerging into the open:

> The pulse, the urine, the sweat, all have sworn to say nothing, to give no indication of any dangerous sickness. My forces are not enfeebled, I find no decay in my strength … I find no false apprehensions to work upon mine understanding; and yet [I] see that invisibly, and I feel that insensibly, the disease prevails. The disease hath established a kingdom, an empire in me[.]

To see the invisible, to feel the insensible: this is the strange and barely defensible sensibility with which the hypochondriac finds themselves possessed. It is the form of insight that Lucy Snowe enjoys when, under the influence of 'that strangest spectre,' she can see what for others is 'wholly invisible.' Or that I would be left with each time the euphoria of the negative test result had worn off. In the absence of any objective evidence, and perhaps without much subjective evidence, one feels. One knows.

Some time ago while riding the tube, I came across an advertisement that stood out among the familiar roster of ads for nutritional supplements and blended Tennessee whiskey. Unfolding across several posters, it went like this: 'Explore risks that may be common in your family tree.' 'See how DNA affects your health.' 'Put your worries to the test.'

The advertisement was clearly suggesting that the knowledge it sold would be beneficial to the customer, although why and in what ways were questions on which it demurred: not mitigate or minimize but 'explore' risks. The claim seemed to be that knowing about one's genetic predispositions to disease would be inherently good. Knowledge itself would be improving. Yes, I thought. I could see myself doing that, in the spirit of exploration.

*

In *Being Mortal*, Atul Gawande observes that 'without the intervention of modern medicine, with its scans to diagnose problems early and its treatment to extend life, the interval between recognizing that you had a life-threatening ailment and dying was commonly a matter of days or weeks.' Today this brief, calamitous death has become the exception, as death typically occurs after a long, uncertain struggle with an ultimately fatal condition which might have been diagnosed years, potentially many years, before its final stages.

Gawande's point is that, by extending the interval between diagnosis and death, advances in screening and detection have transformed the way that we die. However, they have also transformed the way that we live. What better illustration of this could there be than the category of the 'previvor,' the person who is discovered to be genetically predisposed to a disease that they do not (yet) have. Such people are not sick, they don't have any disease, yet from the moment they become conscious of their condition it would not be exactly right to call them 'well.' Some join patient support groups, while others undergo preventive surgery. Even those who don't take such measures will be likely to pay significantly more attention to their bodies, as physical changes and sensations acquire portentous new subtexts.

The term 'previvor' was coined in 2000 to describe the condition of people who are discovered to have a genetic mutation to one of the BRCA genes, increasing their chances of developing breast and ovarian cancer by up to 72 percent and 44 percent respectively. Where some of these people had begun to describe themselves as 'survivors,' there was a perception among some of those in online cancer communities that this was offensive to those who had actually had the disease. Another term was needed, then, one that would better capture the status of those occupying this new middle position between health and illness (it should be noted, however, that for similar reasons the term 'previvor' remains shrouded in controversy).

Having a genetic predisposition to cancer does not mean that one has a disease (or indeed that one will develop one) and it does not produce any symptoms. In this sense, previvorship is an entirely epistemological condition, in which what one benefits or suffers from is a certain form of knowledge about one's body. According to one company offering genetic testing, 'The knowledge that they could develop cancer leaves previvors with three main options to manage their risk – monitoring, medications and risk-reducing surgeries.' What the test does not leave people with are possibilities of not-knowing:

you can choose to ignore what you know, but you can't choose to be innocent of it. Such knowledge forces a decision in the sense that, as soon as one learns that one is genetically predisposed, not deciding to act on this knowledge itself becomes a decision, and potentially a drastic one.

Havi Carel writes about the condition of doubt to which chronic illness can consign its sufferers: 'In bodily doubt we may even worry about aspects of our body that are normally invisible (e.g. liver function) and alter our behaviour accordingly.' Far from alleviating doubt, improved knowledge of our bodies can intensify it by creating new areas for concern: 'Merely knowing about a particular risk associated with illness, whether real or imagined, is often enough to modify bodily habits so they are slower, more hesitant, or otherwise censored.' For Carel this breakdown of the tacit certainty underpinning one's lifeworld can be experienced as an irreversible 'loss of innocence.'

Carel is writing about the sufferers of serious illness, yet, without collapsing distinctions between radically divergent forms of experience, the category of the previvor reveals the increasingly unsteady boundary between the normal and the pathological, the grey zones that have emerged between these two states.

In recent years this boundary is becoming even more blurred, with the rise of consumer genetic testing being offered by companies such as 23andme ('Because you're never done being healthy'). The information provided by consumer-testing companies is often spurious – because the testing itself is inaccurate, is presented with misleading context, or has little practicable predictive value. However, as Carel points out, a feeling of risk, even imagined risk, can effect profound changes at an embodied level. For many, the likely outcome is that these tests will make the future seem more uncertain, increasing levels of anxiety (and so it may, in this regard, be reassuring to know that according to the company's website 23andme can determine your 'Genetic likelihood of developing anxiety').

Far from more precisely isolating disease, advances in screening and diagnostics can in fact serve to push illness further into ordinary life by detaching it from the experience of feeling, or even being, unwell. Writing at the height of the AIDS crisis, Susan Sontag describes how biomedical testing has led to a 'radical expansion of the notion of illness' and the creation of a new category of subject, 'the future ill.' As with syphilis before it, its long latency is what made AIDS so terrifying to those at most risk, the condition's compatibility with states of apparent health. 'A cancer that would hit only homosexuals, no, that's too good to be true, I could just die laughing!' Hervé Guibert has his friend Muzil (a barely fictionalized Michel Foucault) say in *To The Friend Who Did Not Save My Life*. 'As it happened,' he adds, 'Muzil was already infected with the retrovirus, since its latent period … is now known to be about six years.' In the novel and in the journals that precede it, Guibert makes no secret of his own hypochondria, which is to say the rational fear of the sexually active homosexual male in the 1980s, and in both, he unsparingly details the psychic state of being pre-afflicted by an illness that was claiming millions of lives while politicians looked away.

In *Blood Matters*, the journalist Masha Gessen describes the experience of discovering they had the BRCA mutation as that of entering into a new 'society' in which 'people become privy to the information contained in their genes and reshape their bodies – and their fates – accordingly.' And yet, writes Gessen, as screening technologies continue to encroach into daily life, this perhaps anticipates a world to come: the 'rules by which this society lives are an approximation ... of the rules by which my daughter's generation will run its life.' Many carriers of BRCA genetic mutations will, like Gessen, decide to have preventive surgeries, but a less aggressive strategy of 'watchful waiting' is adopted by up to half. Perhaps we can say, then, that the previvor occupies a sort of waiting room. And yet, as Gessen suggests, in an age of genetic testing, early detection, and responsible self-scrutiny, this is the waiting room to which we are all increasingly confined.

*

Hypochondria is the dream of perfect knowledge. What haunts the hypochondriac is everything that remains out of sight, which refuses to remain out of mind. It's as if the hypochondriac wishes to conquer the regions of the latent, so as to absorb them into the manifest; and in this way 'Where it was, there I will be' – Freud's famous dictum about psychoanalysis – could be the hypochondriac's battle cry.

According to the philosopher Peter Sloterdijk, assaults on latency have become the most defining feature of the modern world. In the third volume of his 'Spheres' trilogy – a towering philosophical history of the West – Sloterdijk argues that modernity is defined by 'explication,' a process by which the background conditions that sustain life are thematized and brought to light. As this occurs, what had passed unnoticed is revealed in all its previously unimagined complexity.

Explication has what pharmacists call 'paradoxical effects.' On the one hand explication increases our technical mastery over the environment; yet it also brings with it a sense of our vulnerability, revealing our dependence on atmospheric conditions that are beyond our control. Nowhere, argues Sloterdijk, are the effects of explication felt more acutely than with the atmosphere itself, Earth's main 'life support system,' a necessary condition for a liveable planet. There is less air than you might think: three quarters of Earth's atmosphere sits within eleven kilometres of the surface, after which it rapidly thins, vanishing by degrees into lifeless space, with no definite boundary separating abundance from nullity. Once the undifferentiated medium of existence, air has in recent centuries been shown to be a complex mixture of gases, subject to countless fluctuations, which the toxic effluvia of extractive capitalism are making incrementally less capable of supporting human life. No longer a boundless resource, breathable air is an increasingly scarce commodity. Hence the title of Sloterdijk's long narrative about explication when it was published as a standalone book: *Terror from the Air*.

What really interests me about Sloterdijk's argument is this: far from steadily eroding the regions of latency, replacing hazy ignorance with solid facts, explication in fact serves to generate new latencies. As previously unexpected areas of complexity are revealed, thoughts and suspicions loom about what else remains to be brought to light. Where previously there had been nothing at all, now there are depths waiting to be plumbed. In a further turn, these suspicions are themselves recruited to support further assaults on latency, thus feeding a paranoid and potentially endless cycle: 'Modernity as background explication remains trapped in a phobic circle,' Sloterdijk writes. 'By striving to overcome fear through fear-producing technology, it ... justifies the further use of latency-breaking and background controlling violence.'

In Sloterdijk's description, it's as if there's something hypo-chondriacal about the entire project of modernity. When it comes to individual health, what this points to is the potentially self-defeating nature of the compulsion to know. Afraid I had some form of blood or lymph cancer, I frequently visited the doctor in the hope that testing would put my mind at ease. The thinking behind this was not unreasonable: if I did have the feared illness, there was a chance it would reveal itself when the doctor did my bloodwork; conversely, if my bloodwork or whatever came back as normal, then this would suggest my fears were unfounded, that I was fine. However, in practice things tended to go quite differently, as chemicals and biomarkers that previously I hadn't heard of became new material for concern (bone density low? creatinine high? overall white cell count normal but neutrophils low?). Any anomalies would be submitted to further research online, but these explo-rations tended to turn up more questions than answers, ques-tions that I would later put to the doctor, whose learned response always risked generating new mysteries.

Lately across London I've been seeing posters for a company called Randox Health that say KNOW YOUR RISK and THE POWER TO EXTEND YOUR LIFE, thus putting a new twist on the adage, variously attributed to Bacon and Hobbes, that knowledge is power. Different packages measure different biomarkers ('data points'), 150 to 350 of them depending on the cost. Seeing these kinds of adverts, I become briefly grateful that I can't afford private healthcare. After all, despite the website's promise of 'empowerment' through self-knowledge, isn't there the likelihood that these tests will reveal painful gaps in one's knowledge of their body, gaps that further testing promises to fill?

The problem, surely, is that there is nothing very 'human' about the inside of the human body, with its dark surfaces and occult functions. To what extent can I be said to 'be' my creatinine levels or my kidney function? While current wisdom has extended the logic of individualism by speaking of the uniqueness of each person's gut microbiome, no one who has a colonoscopy ever finds much ground for identification there.

The philosopher Emmanuel Levinas draws attention to this by positing the primacy of the accusative ('me') over the nominative ('I'). Through this distinction he is pointing to the aspects of existence that cannot be fully territorialized, the sheer it-ness of our bodies. For Levinas the linguistic figure appropriate to describing these bare, and barely human, aspects of existence is the impersonal, otherwise known as the meteorological, verb form: 'it rains.' Our lives are sustained by atmospheres and background processes that rarely rupture the surface of attention. With each intake of breath our bodies are flooded by twenty-five sextillion molecules of air, which is to say a mixture of gases and dust, of pollen, particulate matter, bacteria, viruses, protozoa, the tiny airborne organisms that are sometimes called aerial plankton, spores, microplastics and countless other things, natural and humanmade, that we accept into our bodies without ever learning their names. Our skin is constantly falling off at a rate of thirty thousand cells a minute. A million of our cells die each second, more than a kilogram a day. Your body weight every few months. What is that supposed to feel like? Clearly, these things concern me, but where, among all this, am 'I'?

When we feel unwell, it's common to say, 'I don't quite feel myself,' as if to suggest that the increased bodily awareness that even mild illness provokes is enough to rob us of our feeling of personal identity. This is what is wrong with the hypochondriac's dream of keeping the whole body in mind. Feeling well – feeling 'ourselves' – may ultimately rely just as much on what we don't know; or as Sloterdijk would put it, on the implicit. Far from shoring up an empowering sense of health, security, and identity, increased knowledge of one's body can serve to keep one trapped inside a phobic circle, reactivating Cartesian suspicions in which the self is trapped inside an alien entity from which it is fundamentally estranged. Those wishing to attain peace of mind through physical self-knowledge are often led in quite a different direction, such that for those pursuing this path it may ultimately become necessary to invert the Freudian dictum: where I was, there it will be.

THE POWER OF NAMING

If you overlook some of its idiosyncrasies, the situation described by the fairy-tale 'Rumpelstiltskin' is quite familiar: on a day that begins like any other, a woman's darkest fears are suddenly realized. And, worst of all: it all unfolds exactly as she knew it would.

The queen has been living in denial. In a moment of desperation a year earlier, she made a pact with a sprite: he saved her life, and in return she promised to give him her firstborn child. Now he has arrived to collect his prize. Seeing the queen's distress, the sprite agrees to a deal: if she can guess his name within three days, the earlier pact will be annulled. Having made several unsuccessful guesses, the queen (or in some versions her servant) wanders into the woods, coming across a cottage where she spies the incautious stranger singing to himself, 'The queen will never win the game, for Rumpelstiltskin is my name.' The following day she utters his name and, depending on the version, the defeated Rumpelstiltskin either flees the scene or in his rage tears himself in two.

At times there have been names that have held an almost supernatural power over me, names whose simple mention could elicit a bodily response, like the exhilarated, nauseated feeling I experienced one rainy afternoon when, finding myself in central London with an hour to kill, I wandered into the Tate where I was confronted by words (they belong to the artist Ed Atkins) that felt as though they were addressed to me personally: READING THIS TEXT WILL CONJURE A TUMOUR UP INSIDE YOU.

Hypochondria appears to have a special relationship with such acts of naming. It is, writes Elias Canetti, a form of 'Angst which, for its distraction, seeks names and finds them.' 'Naming,' the psychoanalyst Darian Leader tells us, is 'one of the cardinal features of the hypochondriac's experience ... Naming a suspected illness can bring relief to some and intolerable anxiety to others, but the shadow of a name is almost always present in the hypochondriacal complaint.' Where many people are content to be namelessly sick, hypochondriacs tend to be heavily invested in the idea that their suffering is caused by a single, identifiable disease.

Of course such acts of naming can confer practical advantages. Naming, in the form of medical diagnosis, can clear the way for treatment. Moreover it can give the subjective experience of suffering a social reality; it can legitimize suffering, authorize it, and in societies organized around the imperatives of productivity, this can open access to state benefits while normalizing otherwise non-normative behaviours such as absence from the labour market.

But as 'Rumpelstiltskin' suggests, there is a touch of magic in naming, an element of fantasy that is not exhausted by these reasonable explanations. For me, medical diagnosis constituted nothing less than salvation. And while the specific identity of the disease was liable to change – morphing sometime in my early twenties from a brain tumour to Hodgkin lymphoma – the rules of my situation always remained exactly the same: if I could just reveal the secret name before it was too late, then I would be saved.

*

In the WHO's ICD diagnostic manual, naming is elevated to one of hypochondria's essential features:

A persistent belief, of at least six months' duration, of
the presence of a maximum of two serious physical
diseases (of which at least one must be specifically
named by the patient).

Darian Leader has pointed out the tortured logic at play in the
WHO definition. If you can name three diseases, then you no
longer have hypochondria. Meanwhile, if hypochondria is
included in the ICD, then it must be an illness. So, if the patient
can name two illness, and the doctor on this basis diagnoses
hypochondria, then the patient now has at least three illnesses:
'And hence is no longer, by this definition, hypochondriac!
Hypochondria becomes the only illness where the diagnosis
itself is the cure.' Leader is right to suggest that this reveals how
'textbook definitions aim at a pseudo-scientific precision which
is ultimately at odds with the experience of pain.' But what
really interests me is how this hypochondriac dream about
naming finds itself repeated in the clinical definition, as though
to suggest that, for all their antagonism, hypochondriac and
doctor are labouring under a collective fantasy.

Naming has long been valorized in the West. In Genesis,
Adam's first act is to name the animals. They are paraded in
front of him, and, as the New King James has it, 'whatever
Adam called each living creature, that was its name.' In its original context, this is a minor episode, barely a few lines. In the
Middle Ages there was a little scholastic murmuring over all
this (did Adam invent the names, or did he intuit them?) but it
was during the Enlightenment, when the West started to invent
vast taxonomies to objectify and organize all lifeforms – while
increasingly placing white Europeans at the top – that this story
gained new importance, becoming a sort of primal scene for

Western fantasies of epistemological mastery. At the beginning of this period, the philosopher Francis Bacon sounded prophetic when he declared, 'Whensoever he shall be able to call the creatures by their true names he shall again command them.' In later references, this is presented as a *fait accompli*. Here is John Milton's seventeenth-century figuring of this scene:

> As thus he spake, each Bird and Beast behold,
> Approaching two by two, these cowring low
> with blandishment, each Bird stoop'd on his wing.
> I nam'd them, as they pass'd, and understood
> Thir nature, with such knowledge God endu'd
> My sudden apprehension.

In a rendering by Jan Brueghel the Younger, Adam stands in a forest clearing while a pair of lions lie supplicant at his feet. In such depictions the connection between naming, knowledge, and domination is made clear: nature bows and cowers before an intelligence that names it and, in doing so, masters it.

When Carl Linnaeus founded modern botany with his 1735 *Systema Naturae*, he was often called 'the second Adam.' Initially this name was given him with a touch of shade by his rival Albrecht von Haller, but Linnaeus wore it with pride: a frontispiece to the 1760 edition of the book depicts him at work in the Garden of Eden. In Linnaeus's binomial system, species are identified by two names: a generic name (genus) and a specific name (species). Despite the biblical image, the success of this system had a more worldly origin: as Amitav Ghosh has pointed out, it was the result of a political decision, made in the middle of the eighteenth century by the Spanish Empire, that it be used on all its botanical expeditions so that they would share a consistent language. Nevertheless, for Linnaeus and the science he founded, naming had what Donna Haraway calls 'a secular sacred function,' which, she explains, in the context of European expansion created a new type of subject for 'whom inscribing the body of nature gives assurance of his mastery.'

*

'There are more sicknesses than names,' Donne wrote in 1624. The same could probably not have been said a century later, and certainly not by the end of the nineteenth century. The final decades of nineteenth century saw the vast expansion of nosography, the systematic naming and description of diseases, and it was at this time that the Garden welcomed some of its smallest new inhabitants, named according to Linnaean principles: *Mycobacterium tuberculosis*, *Vibrio cholerae*, *Bacillus anthracis*.

In the emerging field of mental medicine, however, the nominative impulse was not kept in check by the existence of morphologically discrete organisms. Names proliferated, typically with classical etymologies so as to confer a touch of officialdom – a situation that the critic David Trotter calls 'taxonomic fury,' pointing to how a practice intended to create order often got out of hand. At the start of the twentieth century the pioneering American psychologist Granville Stanley Hall catalogued a total of one hundred and thirty-two phobic illnesses, from acerophobia (the fear of sourness) to zoophobia (the fear of animals) – stamping each of these new diseases, wrote Freud a little meanly, with 'the magnificence of Greek names.'

Invoking Adam, Blanchot tells us that 'all poets whose theme is the essence of poetry have felt that the act of naming is disquieting and marvelous.' But the Adamic fantasy has held no lesser sway over the scientific imagination (if only pretenders to the role would stop neologizing – or, more likely, if imperial might would once again intervene). In a eulogy for Jean-Martin Charcot, Freud wrote of his former teacher's passion for nosography, and said that the pupil who followed him through the wards of the Salpêtrière 'would recall the myth of Adam … when God brought the creatures of Paradise before him to be distinguished and named.'

As the nineteenth century draws to a close, Freud looks back on those days spent with his former teacher as an Edenic moment when intuition is indistinguishable from invention. By 1910, however, his mind is firmly on the future. Addressing the second Psycho-Analytical Congress with a paper titled 'The Future Prospects of Psycho-analytic Therapy,' Freud sets out his utopian vision of a society emancipated from mental illness, and as he does so, he draws on another literary tradition about naming. When it comes to mental illnesses, he says, their 'capacity to exist depends on this distortion and disguise' and so once 'the riddle they hold is solved and the solution accepted by the sufferers these diseases will no longer be able to exist.' The situation, says Freud, who is evidently thinking of the Grimms' odd little sprite, is the same as 'in fairy-tales [where] you hear of evil spirits whose power is broken when you can tell them their name which they have kept secret.' In this paper, whose humdrum title belies its wild and phantasmatic content, Freud describes naming as a powerful kind of speech that will liberate all of humanity from the curse of disease.

Isn't this the disquieting and marvellous power to which the hypochondriac wants to lay hold? In an age bloated on discourse, naming recalls us to the earliest contract between word and world, a paradise lost. According to Genesis, universal confusion has governed conversation ever since humans, who originally understood each other perfectly and spoke a single language, tried to build a tower to the heavens so that God, in his wrath, scattered them across the face of the earth. To this day we labour under the effects of this divine punishment, the ambiguity it unleashed, whose positive aspect, we might say, is poetry. The oldest surviving philosophical fragment, attributed to Anaximander, is barely thirty words in length; today people read those words and reread them, still trying to determine what they mean – a situation that is helped, or hampered, by the many thousands of words that Martin Heidegger and others have written trying to understand them.

Isn't it weird, when one thinks about it, and disconcerting, that the patient–doctor interactions from which diagnoses emerge are carried out in the same medium as poetry: language, with its endless possibilities for distortion and disguise. 'So, what's the matter?' That simple question, and the room suddenly a blur; then comes the terrible moment when, your own voice echoing in your ears, you hear yourself prattling on, veering way off script, saying all the wrong things. At moments such as these, language, the very thing that enables communication, comes to seem like its greatest impediment.

In the face of all this, the name is like an ideal language that promises to concentrate the diffuse reality of suffering to a single point, to contain it, and make it available for the communication on which action depends. O Lord, deliver us from reading. The fantasy of the name is that of a language that has been shorn of its discursive function, reduced to pure reference. It is the fantasy of standing in the Garden of Eden, unburdened by history or interpretation, bringing the world to heel using nothing more than one's voice.

*

'To him who waits, all things come!' On the face of it, Alice James's pronouncement could hardly have been further from the truth, it being a well-known fact that the overwhelming majority of desires go unfulfilled, and that waiting for some future happiness, as James seemed always to be doing, is the surest (if not the quickest) path to disappointment. 'My aspirations may have been eccentric,' concedes James in the same diary entry; but now that Sir Andrew Clark had diagnosed the lump in her breast, anyone would have to admit them 'brilliantly fulfilled.'

It was an unusual response to a diagnosis of breast cancer. But since her first breakdown at the age of nineteen, Alice James's life could be said to have been a rehearsal for this moment. By the age of twenty-nine, her mother could wearily refer to a complete mental and physical collapse as 'an aggravated recurrence of her old troubles.' And by now, at the age of forty-two, James had spent more than two decades mostly confined to her bed; when she left the house, it was generally in a Bath chair. Her friend (and possibly lover) Katharine Loring would wheel her around Hampstead, Hyde Park, or Leamington for a little airing, then she'd bring her home and play amanuensis as James dictated her next diary entry.

As debilitating as they were, however, James's symptoms could also be maddeningly diffuse: they came and went, waxed and waned, and they rarely left a trace. They had little social reality, which made James vulnerable to suspicions of malingering, or at least of bringing things on herself. Like her more famous brothers, William and Henry, Alice was rarely spared the attentions of headaches, insomnia, and anxiety. But where her brothers dabbled, Alice excelled. Mysterious pains surged through her legs, which regularly failed to work at all. Her heart raced – which might have been worry, or a sign of the Bright's disease that was in the family.

If the James children needed to learn how to be nervous, they didn't have to look far. Their father describes how one evening after dinner, 'fear came upon me, and trembling … To all appearance it was a perfectly insane and abject terror, without ostensible cause.' However, Henry Sr. could discern the presence of 'some damnèd shape squatting invisible to me within the precincts of the room, and raying out from his fetid personality influences fatal to life.' The event, he wrote, 'reduced me from a state of firm, vigorous, joyful manhood to one of almost helpless infancy,' and for years to come its after-effects were to be felt, in ways spoken and unspeakable, by every member of the James household, including those who, like Alice, had not been born yet. In such a familial context, William's self-diagnosed 'philosophical hypochondria' could be written off as a professional hazard, while a touch of nervousness hardly unbecame the author of *The Turn of the Screw*. Alice was in this regard the true prodigy of the family. She devoted herself wholeheartedly to her maladies, and the finest medics of the day were genuinely baffled.

There is power in naming, but who holds that power – how it is distributed between namer and named – is rarely straightforward. The medical gaze can be nullifying, but in a culture that values it, being overlooked can be worse. For decades that had been Alice's fate:

> Ever since I have been ill, I have longed and longed for some palpable disease, no matter how conventionally dreadful a label it might have, but I was driven back to stagger alone under the monstrous mass of subjective sensations, which that sympathetic being 'the medical man' had no higher inspiration than to assure me I was personally responsible for.

What could be more palpable, and more conventionally dreadful, than a cancerous tumour – especially one that (it would be confirmed a few weeks later) had already begun to metastasize? Neurasthenia, hysteria, rheumatic gout, suppressed gout, cardiac complication, spinal neurosis, nervous hyperesthesia, and (which might come nearest to the truth) spiritual crisis: an ever-changing list of names, diagnosed by various doctors, that had done nothing to validate a form of suffering whose most awful quality was its invisibility, its barely being anything at all. Cancer, though. That was something.

A year before Alice's diagnosis, William sent her a copy of his article arguing that the hysteric portions off a part of her consciousness. Alice agreed with her brother's analysis, but writing in her diary, she also suggested that in her own case she simply had too much consciousness: would that she could get rid of some of it. 'Conceive of never being without the sense that if you let yourself go for a moment your mechanism will fall into pie and that at some given moment you must abandon it all, let the dykes break and the flood sweep in … 'tis a never-ending fight.' This fight, as she describes it, which appears to be the fight to preserve the boundaries of her self, is at once tireless and strangely immaterial. It has few rewards, only the right to go on existing in the straitened social roles assigned to her: daughter, sister, invalided spinster. In the face of these conditions, the tumour perhaps represented an abandonment to suffering, its concretisation.

As Alice James gave herself over to dying, she called her tumour an 'unholy granite substance in my breast,' a phrase which speaks to its solidity, its unmistakable reality, like the stone that, as Johnson accompanied Boswell to Harwich one hundred and thirty years earlier, he kicked during the famous debate about George Berkeley's subjective idealism: 'I refute it thus!'

This is what we might imagine James saying to all her doubters, to all those who accused her of bringing things on herself. It is what I myself dreamed of one day shouting at all those friends and doctors who thought I was making it up: I refute it thus! Alice James's case is extreme but I suspect that beneath the hypochondriac's fear of the disease there not infrequently lies another fear, unspoken and indecent, contradicting the first and yet no less haunting for all that: this is the fear that the disease does not exist after all, that one has spent one's life worrying, waiting – for nothing.

Since the early modern period, when hypochondria named a physical illness seated in the abdomen, successive theoretical shifts have seen it rendered increasingly ethereal – first it became a nervous disorder, then a psychological one. This led to suspicions of imposture, and the hypochondriac became a discreditable character as the condition ceased to name an illness so much as the imagination, or simulation, of illness where none in fact existed.

Against the grain of these developments, there have been those who have wanted to restore the idea that hypochondria names a 'real' disease. In the 1990s the psychiatrist Brian Fallon observed that hypochondriacs seemed to respond to SSRI medications, and this led him to write, 'New medical perspectives on hypochondria now suggest that hypochondriacs may in fact be physically ill. However, the illness is not a result of the disease they fear but a neurochemical imbalance in the brain.'

In fact this perspective is not particularly new. Something similar was being argued by George Miller Beard, in 1884, when he wrote that hypochondria is 'truly a disease … and should be treated accordingly.' For Beard conferring reality upon hypochondriacal suffering meant granting it medical status, and this in turn meant treating it (in both senses of that term) as a physical disease. In an era when Koch and Pasteur were making headlines as they unveiled the microscopic yet physical basis for a growing number of diseases, nervous medicine struggled to shed the perception of quackery and imposture. Even celebrated practitioners like Beard could sound a little hypochondriac as they proclaimed the physical reality of the illnesses they treated:

It must be confessed that a large number of cases of chronic diseases are frequently dependent on or connected with some important lesions, of which, during the lifetime of the patient, even the most approved methods of diagnosis and the most practised skill utterly fail to ascertain either the nature or the locality. This is oftentimes the case with … hypochondriasis.

For many it little mattered that hypochondriac lesions could not be found. They were probably tiny anyway, and why go cutting up corpses in search of what even the newest medical instruments were still too crude to detect? All that mattered was that these lesions be postulated, and then hypochondria would be a real illness worthy of a real doctor. After all, what most patients wanted was just to feel they were being heard by the relevant authority. Many years later Jacques Lacan would argue that the attention and counsel of someone whom the culture had elected healer was enough in itself to initiate the work of therapy: 'As soon as the subject who is supposed to know exists somewhere there is transference.' In this era before the advent of psychogenetic illnesses, talking cures, and social-ized medicine, doctor and patient find themselves with over-lapping interests: both require a pretext for their mutually beneficial coming together.

'I wanted my condition to be true,' writes Jenny Diski of her childhood hypochondria. 'Only things with names were real. Fantasy suffering wouldn't do, I ached for authentic suffer-ing.' Perhaps what really matters, then, is not whether hypo-chondria is a 'real' disease, but rather our ideas of the real, our fantasies about reality, and what these things can do to our suffering. From a patient's perspective, one thing that diagnosis can do is create a little space between the sufferer and their suffering; for some this can be a large enough space from which to conduct a life. This is what Alice James is pointing to when she writes that, before her breast cancer diagnosis, she was held responsible for her suffering; afterwards she could settle into the socially accredited role of the patient. With diagnosis my suffering ceases to be entirely 'mine' and becomes a particular instance, a 'case,' that participates in something more general. I have friends for whom this has been nothing less than liberating.

And what about hypochondria itself? In the 1990s, a century after Beard's intervention, the journalist Carla Cantor committed herself to nothing less than 'shattering the myth of hypochondria,' the subtitle of the book she co-wrote with Fallon. Cantor describes the experience of coming across an article about hypochondria in the *New York Times*: 'Suddenly something clicked for me … There *was* something wrong with me, but not a deadly disease … That meant I had nothing to be ashamed of. It meant I could get well.' Such well-meaning efforts may be revitalized by a 2023 study out of Sweden which, comparing the health outcomes of forty-five thousand hypo-chondriac and non-hypochondriac patients, found that hypo-chondriacs on average die five years earlier ('I told you I was ill'?). The study neatly condenses the recursiveness of hypo-chondria as a fear of illness that is also treated as a form of illness, suggesting that anyone who has health concerns would also do well to exercise a little concern about those concerns, to keep them in check lest they should develop into the full-blown fears that could lead to early death.

As Cantor describes it, having nothing to be ashamed of makes it necessary to have 'something.' I'm reminded here of a comment made by Sedgwick that a new faith in biotechnologies has led to a curious reversal: increasingly it is the belief that a particular trait is biological that triggers fantasies of its transformation, while that which used to be described as 'only cultural,' 'merely constructed,' is met with fatalism. Which is to say that in a culture that has placed its eggs in the basket of the biomedical, it is having a diagnosed physical illness that offers the surest prospects for getting better – something that perhaps can be fulfilled by hypochondria itself insofar as we view it as a neurochemical condition. A set of powerful fantasies operate here about medicine and its ability to alter, enhance, augment, and optimise human realities on the condition that they be physically grounded. That which is psychological, on the other hand, or for which no neurochemical basis can be determined, all this can merely be spoken about – probably at great length, and expense, with someone whose first degree was in literary studies – and most likely without results.

'What would you do if you were cured?' Alfred Adler, one of Freud's early followers, used to ask his patients at the beginning of their first session, just after he had let them set out their problem. They would tell him and then, as told by Adam Phillips, Adler would say, 'Well go and do it, then.' I have an American friend who has diagnosed herself with a difficult-to-diagnose, and therefore woefully underdiagnosed, autoimmune disease precisely to avoid having to answer to Adler's tenderly bullying question. Despite her frequent 'doctor shopping,' no one has yet confirmed the diagnosis. On the other hand, maybe she does have it: half the people who go on to be diagnosed with autoimmune conditions, disproportionately women, are initially written off as hypochondriacs, often for years. Of course it isn't like she is unaware of this fact, either – she is full of statistics, this friend – which is also what makes her symptom, if that's what it is (honestly, I have no idea), so brilliantly selected: faced with these realities, who could make her give it up?

Of course the 'problem' with Adler's existentialist question is that we don't necessarily want liberation. If symptoms are inhibitions, then this is precisely their raison d'être: with the symptom standing guard against realization, I can safely keep on wanting what I want (if only I was cured ..., etc.). This is why at the end of Deborah Levy's *Hot Milk*, once she has been diagnosed with cancer, the previously immobile Rose can (literally) walk away from her hypochondria: she no longer needs it.

Discussing the success of Pasteur's germ theory of disease, Georges Canguilhem writes that its appeal lay in the fact that 'it embodies an ontological representation of sickness. After all,' he writes, 'a germ can be seen ... while we would never be able to see a miasma or an influence. To see an entity is already to foresee an action.' If getting better requires that there be something wrong, and that that something become known, then there is a clear psychological advantage in hypochondria itself being deemed to name a physical disease. What is ironic here is that this fantasy – the fantasy that one's suffering can be identified with a single, ontologically discrete disease entity that can be diagnosed, treated, and cured – is probably what drives many people to hypochondria in its initial, 'innocent,' unironized form; that is, before one has learned to see hypochondria itself as the disease from which they need to be cured.

As feminist critics began pointing out in the late twentieth century, Alice James's fate was similar to that of many women of her generation and class, who were educated only to be excluded from serious intellectual pursuits. This is not to reduce James's suffering to a set of social conditions, but rather to point out that it was probably overdetermined – the result of a miasmic combination of factors that cannot be divorced from politics. Meanwhile in 'Rumpelstiltskin,' the queen is a peasant woman who has been sold to the king by her father. The king locks her in a chamber and forces her to perform impossible feats (spinning straw into gold) under threat of death; and it's only because of the pact she makes with the vexatious imp that she lives to be 'rewarded' by being made queen. And yet the tale asks us to believe that, the evil spirit named and defeated, she has been cured, liberated.

Leader writes, 'If someone complains of ill-health, and you push a bit, they will often come up with the name of what it is they are worried about.' And of course, if you push a bit further you'll possibly find a good deal more as the name, really more of a placeholder, eventually disolves to reveal a set of emotions and experiences that are scarcely articulable, or that can only be articulated with considerable effort and at great length over many hours. This is the work of psychoanalysis, which like every type of reading, might turn out to be never-ending – as every interpretation is liable to be displaced by another, and understanding fully means realizing that no understanding will ever be full.

It's in the face of this kind of uncertainty that you can see the appeal of what the critic Steven Connor has called 'the most strongly locked-in of all the assumptions of medical knowledge, namely the fact that illness comes in the form of distinct and ontologically specific diseases.' Call it underdetermination: as I look back today, I feel quite certain it's what I spent years doing, years during which Adler's question, which really is the question of how to live, what to do, was never definitively cast aside but was made perpetually into a question for tomorrow.

Imaginary illness indeed. Could it be that hypochondria names a solution disguised as a problem?

A few years ago in therapy, an old memory rose up like a soap bubble from wherever old memories are stored. In it I am four, maybe five, and my parents, sister, and I are watching the evening news, which contains a feature about a Chinese herbalist who has become famous for his ability to cure virtually any ailment with his pungent green brews. Despite his renown, the Chinese herbalist's prices have remained low, and his practices exemplarily fair-handed: the doors open at five each morning, at which point the first person in line is invited to enter. Then the second, the third, and so on, one at a time. Those who have not been seen by midday, when the shop closes, are invited to try again tomorrow. By 3 a.m. queues are known to stretch around the block. Sightings of celebrities are common.

At that time my mother had eczema across her face and scalp, eczema so severe her hair had started falling out. We watch attentively and then my father calls for someone to get him a pen and paper. The implements produced, he waits until the camera angle changes to reveal the road name, Little Newport Street, on the side of an adjoining building. Then we do something unprecedented. Instead of going to bed, the four of us jump straight into the car and, driving through the night, speed from our suburb in the southwest of England toward the centre of an unimaginably large city named London.

The spontaneity of this still takes my breath away, I tell my analyst. Something about it implying the provisionality of every plan, the solubility of every routine. Considering it now, at a distance of three decades, still produces a sense of spaciousness that makes the future feel unwritten.

Perhaps it is the idea of health as a joint task that appeals to you, offers my analyst. Health as a shared journey. It's possible, I agree, and as I go on speaking the long forgotten scene sharpens into focus, my words seeming to pull the memory from out of nowhere as it occurs to me just how important it was across the years that followed, this night that a few moments earlier I couldn't recall. Shifting on the couch, I tell my analyst about the adventure of getting in the car while it is dark, the transcendent, warm pleasure of drifting in and out of consciousness as we move, steadfastly, through the night. I always enjoyed that, the gradations of sleep that were offered, for instance, by the sofa. At night I always preferred to remain there, amid TV sounds and ongoing chatter, as opposed to going to a bed that was so absolutist, so dogmatic in its delineation of sleep from wakefulness. I explain the divided feeling of being in that car, familiar from so many other journeys: at once an eagerness to arrive and a desire to suspend, indefinitely, the hiatus.

When I finished speaking there was a long pause, after which my therapist said, 'It sounds like a happy memory.' At which point, surprising myself, I began to cry.

*

The following year my family visited me in London. By that point I had lived there for more than a decade. We wandered about the West End, taking lunch somewhere forgettable, and eventually found ourselves on Little Newport Street. This was not in itself an event. For years I had worked nearby, in a famous bookshop, and I must have walked up and down the street a hundred times. But it was incredible, being there that day. Incredible that we should be standing outside the Chinese herbalist's shop, together, more than a quarter of a century after we had last been there during that momentary break with the ordinary that governed life then. It had moved a few doors down but still had the same name, as my mother was able to recall; the new premises were bigger, the consultants now sat behind computer screens, and, a sign of the times, you could book a test for COVID-19. I started telling my mother how remarkable it seemed, looking back. How strange that after seeing that news report we simply hopped in the car that very evening, driving through the night to London. She smiled vaguely. Didn't we have plans? Did they call in sick to work? Had she taken us out of school?

We were in Leicester Square now. Someone inside a large M&M costume was handing out bags of M&Ms to tourists, while someone else, uncostumed, was sermonizing via megaphone.

No, my mother said finally, that's not how it happened. We went a few days later. Besides, she said, you weren't there. We told you about it afterwards, when we collected you from your grandmother.

ECHOES

If we were to see ourselves how others see us, wrote Alice James in her diary, then 'after one or two convulsive laughs, the game would certainly be up!' James is suggesting that self-knowledge is risky, which is why it can be preferable to hide from oneself, to keep oneself out of the picture. 'Narcissus will live to a ripe old age,' prophesied the blind seer Teiresias – 'provided that he never knows himself.'

Narcissus, the beautiful youth. As Robert Graves tells it, by the time he had 'reached the age of sixteen, his path was strewn with heartlessly rejected lovers of both sexes' – including the mountain nymph Echo. Once a loquacious and talented story-teller, Echo was punished by the goddess Hera for having kept her artfully entertained while Zeus made merry with the other nymphs. By the time she meets Narcissus she can only repeat the last words that somebody else has spoken. Later, having been rejected by Narcissus, she (Graves again) 'spent the rest of her life in lonely glens, pining away for love and mortification, until only her voice remained.'

As the victims pile up, the god Artemis eventually decides to punish Narcissus by having him fall in love with his own reflection; he stares at his reflection in a pool, unable escape or to possess himself. Ultimately, he resolves the unbearable situation by burying a dagger in his breast.

'Alas! Alas!' he says.

'Alas! Alas!' repeats Echo.

The myth of Narcissus has become one of the most popular fables of the modern era; for decades successive generations have loved to hate to find themselves reflected in it. Narcissus is an adaptable tale that can be made to stand in for any number of contemporary ills, including hypochondria.

In his 1914 essay 'On Narcissism: An Introduction,' Freud theorizes that each person is endowed with a finite quantity of sexual energy, libido, which they invest in the objects to which they attach themselves, a process that at its most normative involves the selection of a romantic partner of the opposite sex but that can of course mean many other things besides. Within this libidinal economy, the narcissist is someone who over-invests in his or her own ego. Meanwhile, in a further act of misrecognition, the hypochondriac treats not their ego but their body as the site of libidinal investment.

For Freud narcissism and hypochondria constitute a damming up of libido, a failure to take leave of one's own self. At his most extravagantly and provocatively weird, Freud likens the hypochondriac's body to an engorged sexual organ, swollen with attention. This, he suggests, is exacerbated by states of illness: 'The way in which a lover's feelings, however strong, are banished by bodily ailments, and suddenly replaced by complete indifference, is a theme which has been exploited by comic writers to an appropriate extent.' He adds: 'in the last resort we must begin to love in order not to fall ill.'

Freud is hardly the only person to have suspected that hypo-chondriacs could stand to get over themselves; that their oft-rehearsed worries have a hint of self-involvement: 'He's a maudlin, twaddling, selfish fool, and bores everybody who comes near him about the state of his health,' says Sir Percival of Frederick Fairlie, the outrageously egocentric uncle in *The Woman in White*. Or that love might be the answer: Fairlie, like so many hypochondriac characters, is a bachelor.

But when Freud suggested the hypochondriac 'must begin to love,' he was not simply rehearsing the secular creed that views romantic love as terrestrial salvation; he was reinventing it by prescribing the specific form of love that is psychoanalysis, whose medium is the patient's 'transference love' for the analyst. This is where comedy turns into tragedy, since according to Freud hypochondriacs were, by virtue of their very condition, incurable – incapable of being seduced back into health.

Freud here is at his most fatalistic and self-certain: there are certain patients, narcissists and hypochondriacs, who are too in love with themselves to get better – who refuse to exchange their beloved symptoms for the ordinary unhappiness of romantic love. And yet I wonder whether narcissism, or indeed tragedy, is really the best way of understanding hypochondria. Hypochondria is often a folie à deux, emerging out of the oscillating power relations between patient and carer, a scenario depicted by Deborah Levy's *Hot Milk*; or in Albaret's biography of Proust, in which she tells us that 'for all those years' his bedroom 'was his stage, and in a way it was mine.'

'The treatment for hypochondriasis,' writes Arthur Kleinman, 'includes persuading patients that instead of having the disease they fear they have, they are suffering from a psychiatric disorder.' The word 'persuasion' is chosen advisedly; it reminds us that the patient–doctor scene is always a rhetorical encounter, ideally a dialogue.

The poet Kathryn Maris points out that, far from being aloof, the hypochondriac is often desperate to engage with the Other – specifically the doctor who, they believe, might provide them with the answer they so desperately seek. The hypochondriac, Maris suggests, might in this sense more closely resemble Echo, the thwarted storyteller, who, having been rebuffed by Narcissus, 'lives her remaining life in the woods, and then in caves, deteriorating into a sack of bones with a voice, and finally just a voice – a voice that repeats itself.' Maris is not simply inverting the roles (the doctor as Narcissus); rather she is suggesting that these roles are negotiated in relation, and that they're therefore more tentative and reversible than our contemporary language of narcissism allows. Adam Phillips is making a similar claim when he points out that psychoanalysts never sound more grandiose and omniscient – more narcissistic – than when making diagnoses of narcissism: 'No one,' he writes, 'is more narcissistic than the enemies of narcissism.'

Until 2013, the DSM entries on hypochondriasis included among their criteria a 'deterioration in "doctor–patient" relationships, with frustration and anger on both sides.' A doctor's emotional attitude toward their patient was deemed an essential aspect of the diagnosis, an ambiguity that is encoded into the unofficial but commonly used epithet 'heartsink patients': it is the physician's heart that sinks when the patient walks in, yet it is the patient who receives the label. Obviously, there are questions about power here: who is naming whom? But also: it suggests that hypochondria and narcissism are roles that are never arrived at alone; that are always negotiated between two.

There would be no Narcissus without Echo. And an echo is not always easy to distinguish from its source.

*

In recent years critics have been given to talking about a 'narcissism epidemic.' There is seemingly no contemporary ill that cannot be explained with this rare psychiatric diagnosis. Readers of popular psychology books are encouraged to view their personal and professional relationships as perpetually threatened by a legion of pathologically selfish mothers, bosses, and boyfriends, and to get ahead by learning how to 'manage' them. Psychiatrists take to the pages of the Sunday supplements to explain the shortcoming of politicians by reference to their narcissism; while a liberal commentariat regularly informs its readers (who are thereby invited to view themselves as members of an implied non-narcissistic 'we') that in an age of selfies, auto-fiction, and fervid pop-psychologizing, more or less everyone has become a narcissist.

The narcissist is always someone else, and yet one seems to reveal so much about oneself – about one's desires and fears – when using this word putatively to describe the personality of someone else. After all, the person whom I label a narcissist is typically someone who has refused to give me something I want (respect, a correct tax regime, unconditional love), and so my diagnosis is motivated, at least in part, by my own frustrated desires. What I find interesting here is not the rightness, wrongness, or even the legitimacy of such lay diagnoses, but rather the element of self-revelation – as if whenever we use the word 'narcissist,' we are never quite sure whom we're talking about.

Why has the narcissist become a shape-shifting contemporary villain, a convenient way of condensing a diverse set of fears regarding others? Or: what is gained, emotionally or rhetorically, when we move from a moral to a medical register; when we call some ne'er-do-well partner or president not 'bad,' but 'mad' – a narcissist?

It is a curious feature of the literature that has accrued around narcissistic personality disorder that it is addressed to everyone except those suffering from the illness in question. The self in need of help is not Narcissus but Echo. One of the axioms of this genre is the idea that narcissists simply 'cannot' engage with other people's points of view; that, fundamentally blinkered, they are 'incapable of change.' ('They remain as they are,' as Freud once put it.) In this way, a narcissism diagnosis rigorously separates self from other, and, whether expressed as pity or as censure, puts the blame for some failure of relation or communication squarely on the pathological Other.

The person who has been so diagnosed has effectively been escorted from the conjectural arena: a narcissist, they cannot be otherwise than what they are, and it would be misguided or maddening to try to win them over in argument. So it will come as no surprise that the standard advice for how to 'survive,' 'leave,' 'defeat,' or, more ambiguously, 'deal with' such a person is invariably that one should cease to entertain *their* point of view: disengage.

Perhaps with narcissists it takes one to know one, and it is a common enough view that the self-help genre into which these books fall itself symptomizes, aggravates, or possibly causes widespread self-obsession. This was the view taken by Christopher Lasch in *The Culture of Narcissism* (1979), a book written at the dawn of Thatcherism and Reaganomics, whose success surely owed something to a culture that had come to love gazing at its reflection, even – or especially – when that meant seeing its own blemishes.

In recent years, however, something does seem to have changed in the popular literature about narcissism. The sociologist Zygmunt Bauman once diagnosed a contemporary shift from dreams 'of shared improvement to that of individual survival.' Where plenty have interpreted the world, and where Lasch still dreamed of changing it, the aim in the recent literature of narcissism has typically been restricted to self-preservation. Enumerating the 'warning signs' or 'red flags' of narcissistic personalities, countless books and articles encourage readers to be carefully calculating in their social interactions, to vigorously protect the boundaries of their selves: 'In the pages ahead, you'll learn to spot Extreme Narcissists among your friends, family, and co-workers,' promises one popular book whose subtitle is 'Defending Yourself Against Extreme Narcissists in an All-About-Me Age.' Such books encourage a kind of social hypochondria, in which readers are encouraged to see every Other as source of potential threat.

If the tone of these books is fatalistic then it is hardly depressive, often giving licence to an exhilarating nihilism. And so if for nothing else, the bestselling *Becoming the Narcissist's Nightmare: How to Devalue and Discard the Narcissist While Supplying Yourself* is a book that can surely be celebrated for the way it brings into focus a world-view that, one often hears, is becoming increasingly widespread. If you can't beat them …

A few years ago I found myself walking through the London Borough of Islington. It was one of those days where, for no good reason, one wishes to die. Not to kill oneself, nothing so resolute, simply to not be alive for a while, to sample oblivion.

I had spent the day working fruitlessly in the bright, modernist reading room in which I have been resident for more years than I care to recall and whose security personnel, I am convinced, have come to regard me with polite mirthful suspicion. My wasted efforts had left me feeling dejected. At such moments I tend to walk very quickly, wanting to be lost, and this is why, on this particular afternoon, I found myself walking through Islington.

The reasons to endure London are various. Among them though rarely cited is a public transport system that affords depressives the luxury of being able to pace frantically and without aim safe in the knowledge that, wherever the terminus of our heated peregrinations, we will be conveyed home at only a few pounds' expense within the hour.

As I forked right off Upper Street, wishing only to be as far from home as was possible to venture by foot, I happened across one of those spas where they seal you inside a soundproof, lightless capsule where you float in saline water, warmed to body temperature, in a state of complete sensory deprivation. It seemed to me that this was the closest way the city could cater to my desire to place my life in parentheses, to feel what it would be like to feel nothing, and before long I was being accompanied to the therapy suite by a woman wearing a polo shirt and gym shorts who directed me toward the safety lever and briefed me about 'the protocol.'

To float, writes Roland Barthes, is 'to live in space without tying oneself to a place = the most relaxing position of the body.' The line is from Barthes's year-long lecture course about his impossible desire for states of neutrality, a project that occurred to me as I showered, as instructed, lathering myself with luxurious, patchouli-scented body wash before slipping into the pod. As I closed the lid and shuffled into position, some light, inoffensive music picked up in the background. This would last for ten minutes, I had been told, and would resume five minutes before time was up. Between these two periods I was to relax, to let go completely. Relax, I said to myself as I lay back and started to float. Let go completely.

Lying there, I felt inquisitive in an upbeat sort of a way. The feeling was similar to when one comes across some festivities taking place in a foreign town and, with the boldness of the visitor, sees no reason not to partake. Eventually the music died down.

A few minutes after that I felt the lightest itch. Raising my hand to touch my face, I left it ever-so-slightly damp. I raised my hand again to wipe it dry, before realizing that would only make matters worse. And there it was: the thing was spoiled. There was simply no way I'd be able to get beyond it, that damp patch. Getting out to dry off was out of the question; doing so would completely spoil my relaxing experience whose cost, I now calculated, amounted to one pound per minute.

As time passed, I became hyper-aware of the single drip that was making its way, ever so slowly, down my left cheek. I realized I had made a terrible mistake. It wasn't just the drip. The heavily salted water was irritating my eczema. With no other sounds to drown it out, the usual ringing in my ears turned to a roar. Shapes flashed and shimmered in the darkness overhead. My heart raced, and my mind turned and turned.

All this stood in stark contrast to my desire for a state of sensationlessness, which, come to think of it, was what for many years must have been my working theory of health. This is what every hypochondriac dreams of: a state of physical neutrality in which the body, infallible yet oddly imperceptible, would vanish into the background. Georges Canguilhem calls health as 'life in the silence of the organs.' Here in this pod, my own pulse echoing in my ears, the absence of external stimuli only served to foreground the rowdiness of a body left entirely to its own devices.

I should say that this was not a particularly happy time in my life. For a while now, my serious, scholarly study of hypo-chondria had been going badly. I still had not become a historian. For all my efforts, the Word document titled 'Book' had been sitting on my desktop, failing to get any longer. Worse still, the one titled 'Notes' never ceased to grow. Each time I opened this document, I found to my astonishment that it was full of words I had no recollection of having written: raw information that I had failed to transform into knowledge. This vast document, it seemed to me, had become the main obstacle to my book's completion; far from being the consolidation of my learning, it was yet another thing to read.

For the first time in years I'd stopped sleeping. During the day I'd walk around in a stupor. But no sooner would my head touch the pillow than I'd feel a surge of energy. Each night I would lie there for hours thinking about my internet browser, where hundreds of tabs – tabs nested inside tabs – sat unread. I couldn't make sense of it, couldn't form it into a coherent narrative. I tried to compensate for this by reading more and more. Or else by producing yet more pages of notes, beginning new documents whose auspicious blank whiteness quickly became darkened. Thinking about the chaos I'd unleashed was an intensely physical experience. I felt it in my stomach and on my skin. The only way I could coax myself into sleep was by pledging, with a wink, that the following morning I would finally close every browser tab.

As I lay there, suspended in darkness, my mind fell into its familiar grooves. Then somewhere a voice said: picture Rousseau floating on Lake Geneva. I pictured Jean-Jacques Rousseau, the political philosopher, floating in a small wooden boat on Lake Geneva. The voice said: picture Krapp. I thought of Samuel Beckett's 1958 play, his saddest, in which the protagonist's mind is returned with ruthless precision to the moment decades earlier when he'd shared a rowboat with a now-estranged lover:

> We drifted in among the flags and stuck. The way they went down, sighing, before the stem! (Pause.) I lay down across her with my face in her breasts and my hand on her. We lay there without moving. But under us all moved, and moved us, gently, up and down, and from side to side. (Pause. Krapp's lips move. No sound.) Past midnight. Never knew such silence. The earth might be uninhabited.

And at some point, as I thought about this, and then other things, and then other things, all of it now lost, and without it ever becoming clear exactly when, the situation shifted and reconfigured itself, discomfort edged into pleasure. My skin had settled. My mind too. I was enjoying myself. Or better yet, was only minimally there. I lay there, stupidly content in my plastic pod beside the Essex Road in the London Borough of Islington.

In my mind images came and went. Then an image came that didn't go. In this one I was twentyish, alone in bed, thinking about all the terrible things that were going to happen to me. That is always how I see myself when I think back on those years.

But lying there, something occurred to me that meant that this image of solitary brooding didn't quite add up: throughout this period I almost never spent a night by myself. The fact was obvious enough, but through the distorted story-making of memory it had become startling. It is not as if I had forgotten A., my partner throughout that time. And yet as I lay there it occurred to me that, while I don't think I would have kept my fears from her – the deceit itself would be memorable – I had absolutely no recollection of us discussing them, or what she made of it all, or of her accompanying me to any of my countless hospital appointments, as though all of this occurred in a private world completely separate from the one we shared.

After I had showered and dried, I decided I would call A. out of the blue. I wanted to find out what she remembered about that time, how much she'd known. Well, she laughed, you have to remember that I was working at a CBT clinic at the time, I thought everyone was mentally ill, which is its own form of hypochondria, I suppose, but yes I can remember you worrying about your health, although, I don't know, it was never very clear with you what was a joke and what was serious. I do remember thrusting a leaflet about health anxiety on you one day, it had all these different statements, Never, Sometimes, Always, tick one. You laughed at that, and I'm sure you never filled it out. Did you? No, of course you didn't. Did I know you had a headache? Well, you used to rub your brow a lot, I'd often see you from the corner of my eye and you'd have this pained expression, though I don't remember if we spoke about that.

Or maybe we did – I don't know, I was distracted. You did use to talk a lot about tumours. Sometimes in the morning you would sit up in bed and, panicked, you'd say you could smell burnt toast, could I smell it too? But it was like a joke. Not a joke in the sense of not being serious, or anyway, that wasn't clear, but a joke in terms of how you presented it – a sort of performance. Like you were making yourself into a joke, and I remember thinking, Why does he do that? You always knew the names of diseases and it was a topic you liked to appear knowledgeable about. You also liked diagnosing people and I'm not sure everyone appreciated that. I remember wondering if this was in some way linked to your grandmother's death. Although that can't be right since it started earlier, but I remember, when that happened, wondering how it was going to affect you, although I don't remember if it did. So I must have known something, yes, but I don't think I was worried, not particularly, probably not as much as I should have been, or maybe I'm being too hard on myself. I don't remember you taking any medication so you must have done that in private, or maybe I thought they were vitamins or hayfever tablets. Of course it's possible I'm misremembering. And no, I don't remember you thinking you were going to have a seizure. I remember you slept badly but that was your eczema, or that's what I thought it was, I don't know if we spoke about it. Your tossing and turning kept me awake, too, although I knew it wasn't your fault, and anyway it's not like I was the best sleeper in those days. Honestly, it was quite a dark time. I didn't know who I was. Nor did I especially care to find out. It's painful thinking about it now, I was so isolated, like I was disconnected from everyone, maybe not from you. And although I know it isn't the case, that there were friends, parties, that you were there always, whenever I think back on that time it's as if I can only see myself alone. Alone in my room. I used to sit there and have endless thoughts about how I was going to fail, my exams, I suppose, but more generally as well. For months I had repetitive strain injury – do you remember that? – and it became an obsession, I was always visiting the doctor, trying out different arm casts, although I think now that the pain was imagined, that it was only in my head, that it was about something else. Honestly, back then I didn't have much time for other people's anxieties. Now that I think about it, I was really unwell. I had dropped below forty kilograms, do you remember, and I set myself a rule, if I could at least eat a single banana every day, that would be something, but well quite often I wasn't able to stick to it, and at night I used to lie awake thinking about how little I amounted to. Do you remember?

A silence fell that I think we occupied together. I was back home now, lying in bed. Night had fallen. We ended the call agreeing to see each other in person next time she visited London, and to talk about that period of our lives in more detail. Some months later she phoned. On a bright day in September we met at Spitalfields City Farm and over coffee spoke excitedly but quietly so as not to wake her one-and-half-year-old. Once P. was awake, we took her to see the animals, but couldn't get as far as the goats or donkeys that I wanted to show her for the first time. Fixated on the chickens, she had no interest in anything bigger. By the end of that day P. could say my name, which she pronounced 'Wheel,' and as I watched her charge about the park it struck me as incredible that before long she'd forget this day, and me, as in years to come she would forget almost everything of her early life, so many things yet to happen were already consigned to that fate.

A. and I did not speak about the past that day, and I don't think it occurred to either of us to mention it.

EMERGENCY

One evening I fell sick. I had a fever, and I didn't sleep. Nevertheless, the following morning I felt fine, so I went to work. But that evening the fever came back, this time worse. This cycle continued for a week or two.

At the time, I was an outreach worker for a charity for the elderly. This was during David Cameron's Conservative government, a January. The work involved traipsing the streets of north London to inform its elderly residents of which public services would remain. I was working under the aegis of a new organization whose main funders were the councils in which it operated (in many ways it was, I'd later come to understand, a roundabout form of privatization). I was paid handsomely for this work, but by the hour. What was more, it was seasonal; once temperatures reached double digits, this brief and surprisingly lucrative employment would come to an end.

I quickly adapted my routine to these new realities. I'd get up, without having slept, and put my bedsheets in the washing machine (time delay: seven hours). Then I'd cycle across the river and walk around the council estates of north London, which were now mostly privatized, and knock on some doors. The aim was to speak to a hundred elderly people each day, 'interactions' that I'd later transform into data. Then I'd cycle back to Camberwell. I would move my bedsheets from the washing machine to the dryer, update my spreadsheet, eat dinner, wash up, read something and reinstall the freshly laundered sheets. Then I'd fix myself a drink and sit in bed and wait until, just after 11 p.m. and always before 11:20, the fever began to gather. This proved to be surprisingly sustainable. Then one day I collapsed on the stairs.

I took the following morning off work to visit my GP. It was an expensive visit from the perspective of lost earnings potential.

As usual, Dr. C. was patrician and inscrutable. His body had been trained to be semantically neutral, to give nothing away. As I spoke he nodded patiently, his eyes trained on a spot just above my right shoulder. 'OK,' he said, 'let's have a look at you.' Dr. C. placed a stethoscope on my back in order to listen to my lungs, putting his other hand against my chest to steady himself. His grip tightened, signifying something. He cleared his throat. 'Did you have any plans today, Mr. Rees?'

Dr. C. instructed me to go to the emergency department. They would X-ray me today; it would have to be today. I agreed to go straight there. After I left his office, Dr. C. followed me out into the stairwell and called out, 'Mr. Rees, you will go straight there, won't you?'

At the hospital I explained all this to the triage nurse. I was careful to leave nothing out, but also to make no embellishments. She nodded sympathetically as she took in in every detail: his tightening grip, the atmosphere that hung about the room. His haunted tone as he called out to me across the waiting room. When my narrative was over she handed me a piece of paper and asked me to hand it in at reception. The paper read: 'Feels unwell.'

*

Later that day I had an X-ray. True enough, there was a 'mass' in my lungs. Certainly, it was of some concern. But it was impossible to say how much. Naturally, that would depend on what it was ('An X-ray machine is not a precise instrument, young man'). A long period of waiting followed, interrupted by the women who occasionally appeared to take my blood. I regretted having brought nothing to read.

For many hours I sat there, until eventually a junior doctor appeared to tell me how things stood. The results that had come back were normal. Others would take longer. It was possible that I had a virus of some sort. That would explain the chest X-ray: it would be a lymph node, that was all. On the other hand, there were reasons to doubt it. My white cell count was normal. One would expect it to be raised. This did suggest that something more sinister might be going on, but it was too soon to be jumping to conclusions. Anyway, I wasn't to worry. I was to go now, get some rest. I was to come back tomorrow, when I would report to the Medical Assessment Centre.

*

Honestly, this was not unwelcome. In general, the parameters of any medical investigation are determined by the story that one tells about oneself. When one leaves a doctor's office having been told, after a brief examination, not to worry, that what one had taken to be a concerning symptom is merely one of the ordinary vexations of embodiment – that one is, in a word, healthy – the feeling tends to be reassuring only in the short term. Before long, doubts set in. What if one has failed to give the really essential piece of information? What if the small detail which in the blur of the encounter slipped one's mind, or which, in embarrassment at one's paratactic excesses, one deliberately withheld, what if this detail were the truly important thing, the stray thread which would have enabled the doctor to unweave the veil of health and reveal the sick body beneath?

Such, at least, tended to be my experience. In *King Lear* Cordelia laments, 'I cannot heave my heart into my mouth.' She is referring to her inability to give voice to interiority, to perform a private feeling. A patient must heave their entire body into their mouth. They must rally the forces of intellect in order to give an account of a body whose nature is independent of their ability to account for it in language but whose fate now depends on that ability. There is always more one can say, and if the patient fails to say the correct thing then any reassuring words uttered by the doctor will be worse than null; they will be a lure. And yet giving a good account of oneself, an account which will convince a doctor that one is worthy of their time, a reliable witness to one's own body, is also about knowing what not to say. More really isn't always more. It is a writer's problem: what to put in, leave out. But the stakes are different.

The Medical Assessment Centre promised deliverance from the usual cycle of relief and regret. It promised that medicine's investigations into my body would no longer depend upon my skill as a narrator. At the Medical Assessment Centre I would be reduced to a mute object of medical knowledge, anonymous and transparent like an anatomical drawing. The thought delighted me.

*

When I arrived at the Medical Assessment Centre, I was surprised when the receptionist, whom I had never met, knew my name. Actually, everyone there seemed to know me. Over the course of that morning people of various professions made reference to my 'case.'

I changed into a hospital gown. A nurse came to take some blood and, to my surprise, left a cannula in my arm. 'Oh?' I said. 'Don't worry, Mr. Rees,' she said meaningfully. 'It's for your procedure.' A few minutes later a hospital porter arrived with a wheelchair. 'All right, Mr. Rees, hop in.' It dawned on me that I might actually be a patient. It was an unlovely realization that felt nothing at all like vindication. I declined, politely I believe, and said I was perfectly well enough to walk. The porter appeared offended by this preference, mumbling that he would have to check with the doctor. I nodded that he should do whatever he felt necessary as I gathered my belongings into my rucksack.

The porter returned, bearing no evident resentment, and as we made the short walk to the Imaging Unit he prattled cheerfully about this and that, the weather, his two young children, the extension he was building at his parents' house. When we arrived, he withdrew quickly so that my delayed and oddly inflected 'goodbye' was addressed to his back as he receded through the double doors.

At the IU, I was injected with a coloured dye that made my asshole dilate and passed several times through a noisy, large machine. It was the moment I'd been waiting for, my dream come true. Afterwards I was told (without the offer of a wheelchair) to retrace my steps to the Medical Assessment Centre. I sat around for an hour or two, time now completely lost to me until the kindly, brusque Dr. L. appeared. 'Look, it's going to be a while. Go for a walk, get something to eat. We'll call you when we need you, OK?'

Soon I was sitting in a dimly lit coffee shop holding a book, and after an hour, or some hours, I received the call from Dr. L. His voice now sounded completely different, grave, formal, although it was difficult to know what to make of this since he belonged to a class and a generation whose members still possessed a 'phone voice.'

I sensed that my fate was now known – not to me, but to someone. The facts of the matter had come to light; it only remained for them to be conveyed to me. As I stepped out into the street I had a sudden rush of appreciation for ignorance, which, after many years of wanting desperately to know my own body, I realized could be something more than a mere deficit. Ignorance could have a reality and texture of its own, it could be a state of plenitude and possibility. It was a state in which I'd have liked to abide a little longer, perhaps indefinitely.

The sky was luminous and white. It was one of those overcast days that give one the appalling sensation of living inside a fluorescent light bulb. I thought about walking in the opposite direction to the hospital, to the Thames, perhaps, or to the City, where I rarely ventured, but whose shadowy and impersonal labyrinth of skyscrapers seemed to offer the very opposite of what lay in store for me at the Medical Assessment Centre. I thought about never returning, taking my chances.

As my mind was lost to these thoughts, my legs carried me back to the hospital. It wasn't only that a will to knowledge turned out to be the stronger drive. The pleasures of not knowing are necessarily belated. One can always choose not to know. But ignorance, consciously chosen, is nothing at all like innocence.

*

When I returned, Dr. L. greeted me at the door. He told me to follow him into a private room, his voice still grave. I sat on the bed, he on the lid of a metal bin marked BIOWASTE. On the computer screen were the results of a CT scan: my body, illuminated. I was surprised to find myself not feeling very anxious.

It was not a feeling of calm that came over me, however; only abandonment to the implacable logic of the situation.

Dr. L. was going to cut to the chase. The scan showed precisely what he had hoped it would not show, that all through my body my lymph nodes were enlarged. They were, in Dr. L.'s phrase, 'standing to attention,' although he could not say why. What he was saying was, the image was clear enough. But he could not explain what it meant.

A disease was mentioned whose name had long been prominent in my daydreams and nightmares. In my internet browsing history. Hearing its name said aloud (I think for the first time) felt obscene and electrifying. Infection was mentioned, too, although it was with a tone of regret that Dr. L. reiterated that there was no elevation in my white cell count. It was of some concern that the enlarged nodes were distributed evenly above and beneath my diaphragm. 'That will make it late stage,' I offered. 'The ones that concern me are in your chest,' he said. 'They're very deep.'

That I liked Dr. L. was partly because he always spoke as though enlisting your assistance to some shared task. He started every sentence with an imperative, 'Look,' and ended it with a rhetorical 'OK?' These were obvious affectations, which did not make them less effective; his style made any further questioning feel weirdly pedantic, and in an infantilized desire to impress Dr. L. by matching his matter-of-factness I almost forgot that the topic under discussion was my fate.

'Look, nothing is certain yet. There's still a chance that this is just an infection. In which case, in a couple of weeks you're going to forget all about it. Get on with your life. But in the meantime, we're going to have to do a lot more tests. OK?' I nodded. 'Look, I know all this is frightening. But I can promise that we're going to get to the bottom of this. So, come back here tomorrow at nine and we'll get started. OK?' I nodded.

*

In the fortnight that followed I reported each morning to the Medical Assessment Centre. Sometimes I spent an entire day there, other times it was only a fleeting visit to deposit a little blood en route to north London, whose elderly population awaited further news about what would survive the cutbacks to public expenditure that were reported to be 'swingeing' (one of those words that, everywhere for a short time, one rarely hears afterwards).

Many tests were performed, and aside from ordinary pleasantries I was rarely required to speak. I simply handed myself over. That the fever had gone by this time was not considered a reason to desist; now, and for the very first time, medicine had taken an interest in my body that had nothing to do with my experience of it.

One day I had a fine-needle biopsy to determine whether the cells that had clumped into masses inside my right armpit were cancerous; it would take a week or more for the results to come back. The intervening period was colourless and strange, and the waiting rooms in which I often sat came to seem like a metaphor for life itself.

On the other hand, I was learning a lot. Partly by osmosis – I was spending so much time on the ward – and partly because of the hospital's practice of copying patients in to all correspondence between its consultants and the patient's GP. Due to a time lag of three or four days, these letters would always arrive a little out of sync with where things currently stood. This did not render them an irrelevance, however: addressed not to me but to my GP, they presented information about my case in a way that was novel and strange.

The feeling when reading these letters was similar to over-hearing a conversation about one's behaviour at a recent party. The deviation from one's own memory need not at all be great for it to kill one on the spot. In these curt yet suggestive letters there would frequently be reference to things that had never been discussed with me ('ACE level elevated'; 'liver function abnormalities'; 'inconclusive') while matters which I'd considered settled days earlier were repeatedly thrown back into question. And so while the letters fizzed with information – information that I would supplement with further information drawn from Google searches – I tended to come away from having read them feeling more, not less, in the dark.

When, after a fortnight or so, it was revealed that I'd had glandular fever – this had initially been ruled out on the basis of an antibody test, but showed up on a subsequent test – I was delighted. It was like one of those criminal judgments in which the accused is given some trivial sentence and, having served this time awaiting trial, is free to go.

The feeling did not last, however. On the day the receptionist told me over the phone about the glandular fever result, I was due to report to the Medical Assessment Centre to get the result of the biopsy. I asked the receptionist if I should keep the appointment, now that we had an explanation. She asked me to hold the line while she discussed this with the consultant – a distant murmuring I could hear but not make out – and when she returned told me, emphatically, that I was indeed required to keep the appointment.

At the appointment, however, which so emphatically was necessary, and which I attended with a frank terror I had not experienced in the two weeks hitherto, the consultant said that he was confident that the glandular fever result explained the abnormalities he'd found in my biopsy.

So there were abnormalities in my biopsy?

No, no. Well, not once we take into account the glandular fever. I can tell you, he said with a chuckle, I was happy to see that.

What about my ACE level?

What about it?

It's elevated.

Oh, it is? Hmm.

And my liver function, it's abnormal.

Well, in any case it's nothing to worry about. You're fine, Mr. Rees. The consultant cheerfully handed me a form discharging me from the care of the Medical Assessment Centre. It was his way of asking me to leave.

I had been an outpatient of the Medical Assessment Centre for a fortnight, or thereabouts. Now I was leaving, healthy. At home, letters continued to arrive for several days.

The charity I worked for did not give its casualized staff sick pay, and so I did not rest, as was advised. Quite the opposite, since my recent absences had been expensive. Probably the work did me good. My period of employment ended in the spring.

*

My memories of the period that followed are more knotted, much harder to give an account of. It is when I came closer than I ever have to madness. Following a brief period of remission, doubts set in. There were so many things that did not make sense. I'd kept the correspondence between the hospital and the GP, which, now thumbed and coffee-stained, was full of incongruous details; it seemed to me to provide a lengthy record of leads unpursued.

I started to resemble poor Miss Flite from *Bleak House*, making myself a continual presence at the GP surgery and at the hospital, always, of course, with 'my documents.' There were a good many things that I'd have liked to know, things I would have liked to clear up. A scan, I thought. That would do it. A scan that would light up every region of my body, that would reveal, clearly and distinctly, what was the matter with it. That would require me to enlist the help of doctors. This was a task to which I applied myself vigorously.

It was a dark time, which went on for many months, during which ordinary life, as it is wont, went on too. And then at some point, without ever really concluding, that period of my life ended.

*

Now, I prefer not to know. I rarely visit doctors; my internet browsing history no longer resembles a diagnostic manual. It has been this way for some years. I don't know how this happened exactly; like any transformation in Weltanschauung it had no present tense. It was only possible, afterwards, to observe that I no longer paid much heed to my health. A few years ago I began writing about all this; the fact might be relevant. If I were to become sick now I'd probably be the last to realize. I don't know that this necessarily represents an advance but certainly it has made life pleasanter.

A few weeks ago I noticed a lymph node the size of a conker in my right armpit, and then another. A few days later I visited the doctor, who suggested sending me for an ultrasound. A few days after that, a text message arrived containing a link through which I could book the hospital appointment: the earliest one was four days later, but I could choose from the many available appointments, in various convenient locations, the one that suited me best.

I have not yet booked the appointment, although I have thought of doing so many times. The lymph nodes remain enlarged. I do not feel frightened, but I do continue to put it off. I have been busy, writing. It is only now, in the very final stages of editing this essay, that the thought occurs to me (it is a thought which makes me smile) that these two things – the appointment that I haven't made, and the essay that I have been writing – could be related.

The above narrative was published in a literary magazine a couple of years ago, after I was commissioned by its then editor to write something about illness. By now my serious, scholarly study of hypochondria had fallen apart. I couldn't get my facts straight, get the story right. I mention this because, including this narrative here, I decided to leave the tenses in the final paragraphs ('I do not feel frightened ... '; 'the thought occurs to me ... ') intact, even if that creates a little messiness since the 'essay' is now part of a book, and the 'now' to which it refers is now a 'then.' This is always the way with deictic words, which, as Judith Butler tells us, work 'only by remaining indifferent to [the] occasion,' and therefore by way of a kind of sleight of hand: it is only because 'now' could refer to any moment that it is able to fulfill its illusionary function of grounding the text in this particular moment.

*

I want to supplement this story with a few words more. Once I had submitted my revised copy to the (concerned) editor I immediately booked an ultrasound: the sonographer looked at the enlarged lymph nodes and, for reasons I can't recall, said they were nothing to worry about. I left the hospital with a familiar glad feeling. After the essay was published, it was picked up for syndication by a national newspaper. It didn't garner much notice, but I received a handful of messages by people claiming to be doctors, and at least some of whom did seem to be doctors, imploring me to get another opinion. One woman felt furiously cheated: reading all the way to the end to discover that I only had glandular fever, she said, that was very disappointing. After a few days, the messages stopped.

About a year later, I was at the launch for a book I'd edited. A man entered the bookshop and immediately approached me and said, 'You're Will Rees. You wrote an essay about lymphoma. I see you around. You go to the British Library.' We chatted politely and after a few minutes he said, 'You need to get another test.' He explained that he'd had lymphoma, that he had been reassured by several NHS doctors that he was fine but continued to feel unwell and ultimately that he 'just knew' what it was. Eventually he went to Harley Street where a private physician diagnosed him without delay. Coming across my essay online was unnerving, he said, uncanny, and his first response was, 'This person has lymphoma.' (That I had decided against mentioning this name in the essay made his statement the more alarming, as if it were a diagnosis, though I suppose I'd made the disease identifiable enough.) He had even thought of finding a way to contact me – and now, barely a few weeks later, here I was. It was incredible, he said. He had the name of the doctor. If I wanted, he would put us in touch.

I found the whole thing weird, offish, and attempting to cut things short I explained that, as it happened, I was scheduled for an MRI on my neck the following week. It was a musculo-skeletal thing, just too much time at my desk, but if there was something more insidious it would presumably show up. He asked how long it had taken me to get the referral. A couple of weeks, I said. And with the amused, ironical tone that one sometimes takes with a small child, he said, 'Do you really think NHS doctors send people for scans within a fortnight when they are sure there is nothing to be worried about?'

I don't want to overextend things by going into a lot of detail about that MRI, the panic it induced in me, which till that day I hadn't felt in years, or about other events that occurred later. Instead I want to return to that troublesome 'now,' which, unsmoothed, breaks the surface of this book and gives lie to the illusion that it has come together all at once. If it has come together, it has done so over a long time, it having been written from out of a series of present moments that each had their own uncertainties. As does this one, which for what it's worth is 2 February 2024, just after 9 p.m. – a Friday night, late in the writing process yet no more privileged than any other moment. The problem of occasionality points to something that tends to be occluded when people make and publish stories out of their experiences: the unbridgeable gap between writing and reading, the fact that the self that gets written, and therefore read, necessarily lags behind the self that writes, so that endings, however indefinite, however hedged or reflexive, are always openings onto stories that never get told.

CODA: GETTING BETTER

It was a bright morning, April, not cold out. As I approached the hospital, it occurred to me that today could be momentous and terrible, one of those days that, afterwards, one remembers.

This was a year before the headache began. I had discovered a lump on my right testicle when I was fifteen but was quick to put it out of mind. I suppose it just seemed too outlandish, too disconnected from the flow of events that made up life then. In the years that followed I mostly forgot about it. Occasionally it occurred to me, sometimes prompted by my experiencing a pain there, a dull and empty sort of ache. But this was always at night. I'd lie there and consider my doom before promising myself I would finally pay a visit to the family doctor. Yet somehow, when I woke up the next morning, all mental trace of those midnight vows would have vanished. Then some weeks later, or probably some months, it would come back to me, this time more pressingly – but once again as I lay in bed.

It went on like this for several years. It was only when I was nineteen and now living away from home that I finally saw a doctor, who immediately referred me for an ultrasound while reproaching me, with a vehemence that I was quite startled by, for having waited so long.

Despite this long preface, the scan was over in a couple of minutes: it was avascular, said the sonographer, benign, nothing to worry about.

When I walked out of that hospital, a light breeze was blowing that swept away four years' anxieties like they were dandelion seeds that had got caught on my sleeve. Joy, I suppose, is what you'd call that feeling. A sort of generalized, objectless YES. As if the tide had receded for the first time in years, revealing, in the space that had been opened up, ample conditions for life. If I had any plans that day, I didn't keep them. I walked around the city with a mischievous, brave feeling, not talking to anyone, just quietly enjoying the secret of what had not happened.

This was the first time I had experienced this feeling, though later I'd encounter it again.

*

'There is no health,' Donne once wrote. 'Physicians say that we, / At best, enjoy but a neutrality.' Meanwhile the dictionary says that health is 'the state of being free from illness or injury.' This makes it a negative phenomenon – not a presence but an absence. Maybe this is why the search for health so often leads one toward dark places. Hypochondria might be called phantom illness, but really, health is the experience that haunts.

'It is sickness that makes health pleasant,' wrote Heraclitus, the weeping philosopher, in one of the fragments attributed to him. In the *Republic*, Socrates is quick to dismiss this idea. The sick person believes that in the recovery of the neutral state lies the greatest pleasure. But for the person already in the throes of pleasure, the same state spells its end and thus the start of their suffering. 'What, then, we just now described as the intermediate state between the two – this quietude – will sometimes be both pain and pleasure … Is it really possible for that which is neither to become both?' As Socrates explains to Glaucon, only philosophy can provide true and positive pleasure, whereas getting better, like every non-philosophical pleasure, is merely a temporary relief from suffering.

I wouldn't be so quick to dismiss that quietude that exists between parentheses. Here's how Baudelaire describes the condition of the convalescent: 'He has only recently come back from the shades of death and breathes in with delight all the spores and odours of life; as he has been on the point of forgetting everything, he remembers and passionately wants to remember everything.' For Baudelaire, the experience of getting better instills a new perception, a heightened attention. Having come so close to leaving it, one is able to embrace the world in all its pungent imperfection.

'The convalescent,' Baudelaire writes, 'enjoys to the highest degree the faculty of taking a lively interest in things, even the most trivial in appearance.' By the time he wrote these words, which appear in 'The Painter of Modern Life,' Baudelaire had spent many years adjusting himself to the patterns of secondary syphilis: the appalling crises, the ecstatic periods of reprieve. Grim thoughts about the future. Lately, it had got into his joints.

In his celebration of convalescence, Baudelaire draws heavily on Edgar Allan Poe's story 'The Man of the Crowd.' The story opens with the narrator, newly recovered from an unnamed illness, sitting at the bow window of a coffeehouse and watching the scene outside with a sort of free-floating attention: 'I felt a calm but inquisitive interest in every thing' (I love that division of the final word, lost in some editions but so essential to Poe's meaning: the convalescent imagination as a sensitivity to the particular, a refusal to subsume it under the general). Poe's convalescent has left his sickbed but he has not quite re-entered the social fray; there is a pane of glass separating him from the street, which, he tells us, is one of the 'principal thoroughfares' of London. From his vantage he is hyper-visible yet oddly incognito. When evening comes on a stranger catches his eye; finally he vacates his window seat and spends the night wandering through the city, following this man in a dreamy, half-serious pursuit, taking in all the life that is vibrating around him.

Once you start looking, the convalescent is everywhere in literature, quietly enjoying what is most ordinary. Lying recumbent, Woolf's convalescent discovers the cloud-filled sky in all its majesty. Stricken by illness, Nietzsche's Zarathustra falls into a week-long slumber; when he awakes, the serpent and eagle who have kept vigil over him say, 'Do not speak further, thou convalescent … but go out where the world waiteth for thee like a garden.' A world that has become a garden is one in which every corner, even the remotest and most inhospitable places, are as though purposefully designed for one's enjoyment. Nietzsche knew that feeling. Lou Andreas-Salomé, his friend and interlocutor, and his unrequited love, once noted the cycle of relapse and recovery that lent his life its syncopated beat. Of the moments of convalescence that Nietzsche cherished, and perhaps cultivated, Andreas-Salomé writes: 'All things then become new even to the mind – "neuschmecken" or "new tasting," as he called it.'

After Andreas-Salomé broke off their friendship, Nietzsche fell into one of his worst periods of crisis. When he had returned to health, he reissued *The Gay Science*, now prefacing it with a long paean to the 'intoxication of convalescence': this book, he tells us, 'contains high spirits, unrest, contradiction, and April weather, so that one is constantly reminded of winter's nearness as well as of the *triumph* over winter that is coming, must come, perhaps has already come … ' For Nietzsche, convalescence is not a naive rebirth but 'a more dangerous second innocence'; which is to say that it's the proximity of an unforgettable past that injects novelty into the new.

Against fantasies of complete recovery, convalescence seems to speak to the uncertainties and vicissitudes of any transition from sickness into health. Nietzsche's convalescent is 'ticklish and malicious.' Poe calls convalescence 'the converse of ennui,' as though to suggest both a radical divergence and a sly affinity between the two conditions – an ambivalence also noted by Samuel Taylor Coleridge when he speaks of 'the voluptuous and joy-trembling nerves of convalescence.' Here we're confronted by the intoxicating, and I am tempted to say addictive, pleasures of getting better: it's as though the convalescent is never quite able to say if they are well, only, and emphatically, that they are alive.

*

One of the most frequently occurring motifs is that convalescence produces a sort of atmospheric awareness, what Roland Barthes calls 'consciousness of mist.' 'In good health,' wrote Emerson, 'the air is a cordial of incredible virtue.' Or Poe: 'Merely to breathe was enjoyment.' Or Joan Didion, after the retreat of one of her migraines: 'There is a pleasant convalescent euphoria. I open the windows and feel the air.' To feel the air, the vanishingly thin layer separating life from cosmic nullity. If there is a positive experience of health, then I don't think it's as a long and regular work. Instead I think it's encountered in those fleeting moments when ordinariness is experienced as a sort of miracle, when the background conditions that support life become manifest as a source of pleasure.

What would it mean to live like that? Aldous Huxley once wrote of his consumptive friend D. H. Lawrence that his 'existence was one continuous convalescence; it was as though he were newly reborn from a mortal illness every day of his life.' Here convalescence becomes a permanent state of renewal; as if, under the pressure exerted by the end, one were forever beginning anew, were continually getting better (and better). Baudelaire goes further, detaching the experience of recovery from any specific experience of illness. He asks us to imagine a person 'perpetually in the spiritual state of the convalescent,' an 'eternal convalescent,' as he puts it, as though to speak of a recovery that is endlessly deferred, a potentiality held in suspense, a future that is forever on the cusp of solidifying into a present.

As I search for an ending, I once again find myself thinking back on that brief ultrasound appointment aged nineteen, a year before the headache started. I'm not sure why my mind keeps being drawn back there. What, after all, even happened? Nothing, or nothing important. I walked into the hospital without a serious illness and I left it without one. Nonetheless, everything was changed. Stepping back outside I felt nebulous and powerful – like arriving in a foreign city and feeling you have taken a holiday from the self. The following year I would be back there. After that, other experiences in other hospitals lay in wait. But all that was yet to come. For now, as I wandered through the streets, which were the same streets I walked through every day, only now, it seemed, a little wider, I felt, for a day, or maybe it was only for an hour, as if anything was possible. I felt as if I might live forever. I felt well.

SELECTED BIBLIOGRAPHY

Albaret, Celeste. *Monsieur Proust*. New York Review of Books, 2003.

Barthes, Roland. *S/Z*. John Wiley & Sons, 2009.

———. *The Neutral*. Columbia University Press, 2007.

Beaumont, Matthew. *The Walker: On Finding and Losing Yourself in the Modern City*. Verso Books, 2020.

Beckett, Samuel. *The Complete Dramatic Works of Samuel Beckett*. Faber & Faber, 2012.

———. *Three Novels: Molloy, Malone Dies, The Unnamable*. Grove Press, 2009.

Bell, Matthew. *Melancholia: The Western Malady*. Cambridge University Press, 2014.

Belling, Catherine Francis. *Condition of Doubt: The Meanings of Hypochondria*. Oxford University Press, 2012.

Bergson, Henri. *Laughter: An Essay on the Meaning of the Comic*. Courier Corporation, 2013.

Berlant, Lauren, and Lee Edelman. *Sex, or the Unbearable*. Duke University Press Books, 2013.

Blanchot, Maurice. *The Book to Come*. Translated by Charlotte Mandell. Stanford University Press, 2003.

———. *The Space of Literature*. University of Nebraska Press, 2015.

———. *The Work of Fire*. Translated by Charlotte Mandell. Stanford University Press, 1995.

———. *The Writing of the Disaster*. Translated by Ann Smock. University of Nebraska Press, 1995.

Boswell, James. *Boswell's Column: Being His Seventy Contributions to the London Magazine Under the Pseudonym the Hypochondriack from 1777 to 1783 Here First Printed in Book Form in England*. William Kimber, 1951.

———. *The Life of Samuel Johnson*. Edited by Christopher Hibbert. Penguin Classics, 1979.

Boyer, Anne. *The Undying: A Meditation on Modern Illness*. Penguin, 2020.

Bronte, Charlotte. *Villette*. Penguin Classics, 2004.

Burton, Robert. *The Anatomy Of Melancholy*. New York Review of Books, 2001.

Butler, Judith. *Senses of the Subject*. Fordham University Press, 2015.

Canetti, Elias. *Kafka's Other Trial*. Penguin, 2012.

Canguilhem, Georges. *On the Normal and the Pathological*. D. Riedel Publishing Company, 1978.

Carel, Havi. *Phenomenology of Illness.* Oxford University Press, 2018.

Cioran, E. M. *The Trouble With Being Born.* Penguin UK, 2020.

Collins, Wilkie. *The Woman in White.* William Collins, 2011.

Crary, Jonathan. *24/7: Late Capitalism and the Ends of Sleep.* Verso Books, 2014.

Deleuze, Gilles. *Essays Critical and Clinical.* Verso Books, 1998.

Descartes, René. *Descartes: Meditations on First Philosophy: With Selections from the Objections and Replies.* Cambridge University Press, 2017.

Didion, Joan. *The White Album.* Fourth Estate, 2017.

Dillon, Brian. *Tormented Hope: Nine Hypochondriac Lives.* Penguin, 2010.

Donne, John. *Devotions Upon Emergent Occasions and Death's Duel: With the Life of Dr. John Donne by Izaak Walton.* Knopf Doubleday, 1999.

Ferenczi, Sándor. *First Contributions to Psycho-Analysis.* Routledge, 2018.

Foucault, Michel. *The Birth of the Clinic: An Archaeology of Medical Perception.* Translated by A. M. Sheridan. Routledge Classics, 2003.

Freud, Sigmund. *The Revised Standard Edition of the Complete Psychological Works of Sigmund Freud.* Edited by Mark Solms. Translated by James Strachey. Rowman & Littlefield, 2024.

Gawande, Atul. *Being Mortal: Illness, Medicine and What Matters in the End.* Profile Books, 2015.

Graves, Robert. *The Greek Myths.* Penguin, 2012.

Guibert, Hervé. *To the Friend Who Did Not Save My Life.* Translated by Linda Coverdale. Serpent's Tail, 2021.

Gumbrecht, Hans Ulrich. *After 1945: Latency as Origin of the Present.* Stanford University Press, 2013.

Hazlitt, William. *Metropolitan Writings.* Fyfield Books, 2005.

Huysmans, Joris-Karl. *Against Nature.* Penguin, n.d.

James, Alice. *The Diary of Alice James.* Northeastern University Press, 1999.

Jerome, Jerome K. *Three Men in a Boat and Three Men on the Bummel.* Edited by Geoffrey Harvey. Oxford University Press, 2008.

Kafka, Franz. *Letters to Felice.* Edited by Erich Heller and Jurgen Born. Schocken Books, 1989.

———. *Letters To Milena.* Vintage Classics, 1992.

———. *The Complete Short Stories.* Vintage Classics, 1992.

Kant, Immanuel. *Religion and Rational Theology.* Cambridge University Press, 2001.

Kierkegaard, Soren. *Either/Or: A Fragment of Life.* Penguin UK, 2004.

Kierkegaard, Søren, and Albert Anderson. *The Concept of Anxiety: A Simple Psychologically Orienting Deliberation on the Dogmatic Issue of Hereditary Sin*. Princeton University Press, 1980.

Levy, Deborah. *Hot Milk*. Penguin UK, 2016.

Mann, Thomas, and A. S. Byatt. *The Magic Mountain*. Translated by John E. Woods. Everyman's Library, 2005.

Melville, Herman. *Moby-Dick: Or, The Whale*. Penguin Classics, 2003.

Miller, D. A. *Hidden Hitchcock*. University of Chicago Press, 2016.

Nancy, Jean-Luc. *The Fall of Sleep*. Fordham University Press, 2009.

O'Rourke, Meghan. *The Invisible Kingdom: Reimagining Chronic Illness*. Penguin, 2022.

Phillips, Adam. *On Getting Better*. Penguin UK, 2021.

———. *Promises, Promises*. Faber & Faber, 2016.

Poe, Edgar Allan. *The Penguin Complete Tales and Poems of Edgar Allan Poe*. Viking, 2011.

Santner, Eric L. *On the Psychotheology of Everyday Life: Reflections on Freud and Rosenzweig*. University of Chicago Press, 2007.

Sartre, Jean-Paul. *Being and Nothingness: An Essay on Phenomenological Ontology*. Routledge, 2003.

Scarry, Elaine. *The Body in Pain: The Making and Unmaking of the World*. Oxford University Press, 1988.

Sedgwick, Eve Kosofsky. *Epistemology of the Closet*. University of California Press, 2008.

———. *Tendencies*. Duke University Press, 1993.

———. *Touching Feeling: Affect, Pedagogy, Performativity*. Duke University Press Books, 2003.

Sloterdijk, Peter, Wieland Hoban, Lotringer, and Sylvère. *Foams: Spheres Volume III: Plural Spherology: 3*. Semiotexte, 2016.

Sontag, Susan. *Illness as Metaphor and AIDS and Its Metaphors*. Penguin UK, 2013.

Strouse, Jean. *Alice James: A Biography*. Harvard University Press, 1999.

Tillman, Lynne. *Mothercare*. Peninsula Press, 2023.

Vila-Matas, Enrique. *Mac and His Problem*. Translated by Margaret Jull Costa and Sophie Hughes. Vintage, 2021.

Williams, Bernard, ed. *Nietzsche: The Gay Science: With a Prelude in German Rhymes and an Appendix of Songs*. Cambridge University Press, 2001.

Woolf, Virginia, and Hermione Lee. *On Being Ill*. Paris Press, 2002.

Zizek, Slavoj, Momus, and Audun Mortensen. *Zizek's Jokes*. MIT Press, 2018.

ACKNOWLEDGEMENTS

A stranger once told me I had two speeds: slow and off. Thank you to those whose patience has been tested as I have toggled between them, above all to Alana Wilcox, whose editing has improved this book in many ways.

Thank you, too, to the editors who have commissioned pieces that have informed, and in places formed, *Hypochondria*: Sally Davies, Marina Benjamin, Vanessa Peterson, Alice White, Danny Birchall, Sigrid Rausing, Spencer Quong, Peter Boxall, and Michael Naas.

Thanks to the friends, readers, and interlocutors whose comments, insights, and encouragement have enriched this book: Sam Fisher, Beatriz Salamanca, Josh Cohen, Daisy Lafarge, Fabrice Leveque, Jen Kabat, Kathryn Maris, Amber Husain, Luke Bird, and Holly Connolly. Thank you to Julie Walsh. A special thank you to Susan Ridpath.

Thank you to Matthew Beaumont for his unwavering support, to Matthew Sperling and Stephen Cadywold, and to the Wellcome Trust (especially Tom Bray). Thanks to Akin Akinwumi for seeing something when there wasn't very much there, and to Crystal Sikma and everyone else at Coach House.

Thank you to Jeffrey Zuckerman and Jacob Rogers for their kind efforts with tracking down a copy of Hervé Guibert's journals.

To all the writers whom I've been fortunate enough to edit at Peninsula, and whose thinking has, without exception, reshaped my own: it has been a privilege to be in conversation with you. The same to the following teachers: Tanja Staehler, Paul Davies, Dylan Trigg, and Josh Cohen.

Thank you to my parents, who have never told me not to.

And, very importantly, for shelter at various periods while writing, thank you to Tom Morgan, Ruth Brown, Liam Sabec, Sara Kaeni, Fabrice Leveque, Sarah Anderson, Emma Rees, Adam Klugg, and Eugenia Lapteva.

And thank you to Ana, whose love and whose questions have in countless little ways changed this book, and me.

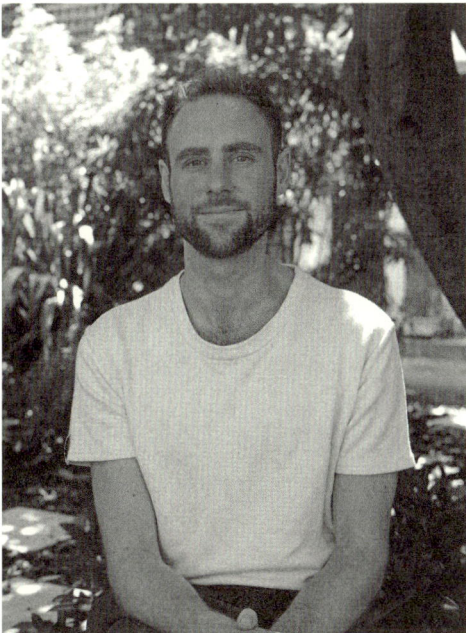

Will Rees is a writer and editor living in London. He is a director of Peninsula Press, which he co-founded in 2018.

Typeset in Arno and Drescher Grotesk BT Bold.

Printed at the Coach House on bpNichol Lane in Toronto, Ontario, on FSC-certified Sustana recycled paper, which was manufactured in Saint-Jérôme, Quebec. This book was printed with vegetable-based ink on a 1973 Heidelberg KORD offset litho press. Its pages were folded on a Baumfolder, gathered by hand, bound on a Sulby Auto-Minabinda, and trimmed on a Polar single-knife cutter.

Coach House is located in Toronto, which is on the traditional territory of many nations, including the Mississaugas of the Credit, the Anishnabeg, the Chippewa, the Haudenosaunee, and the Wendat peoples, and is now home to many diverse First Nations, Inuit, and Métis peoples. We acknowledge that Toronto is covered by Treaty 13 with the Mississaugas of the Credit. We are grateful to live and work on this land.

Edited by Alana Wilcox
Cover design by Luke Bird, cover image by Sean Benesh on Unsplash
Interior design by Crystal Sikma
Author photo by Sophie Davidson

Coach House Books
80 bpNichol Lane
Toronto ON M5S 3J4
Canada

mail@chbooks.com
www.chbooks.com